EVALUATING RESIDENTIAL FACILITIES

ERRATA

Please note the following corrections:

On page 9, the second column heading in Table 1.3 should read: *Domiciliaries (N = 24 Facilities)*.

On page 323, the fourth row of Table E. 2 for *Utilization of Health Services* should read: 9.

EVALUATING
RESIDENTIAL
FACILITIES

The Multiphasic
Environmental
Assessment Procedure

RUDOLF H. MOOS
SONNE LEMKE

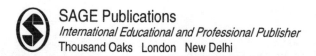
SAGE Publications
International Educational and Professional Publisher
Thousand Oaks London New Delhi

For information address:

SAGE Publications, Inc.
2455 Teller Road
Thousand Oaks, California 91320
E-mail: order@sagepub.com

SAGE Publications Ltd.
6 Bonhill Street
London EC2A 4PU
United Kingdom

SAGE Publications India Pvt. Ltd.
M-32 Market
Greater Kailash I
New Delhi 110048 India

Printed in the United States of America

Library of Congress Cataloging-in-Publication Data

Moos, Rudolf H., 1934-
    Evaluating residential facilities:
The multiphasic environomental assessment procedure / authors, Rudolf
H. Moos, Sonne Lemke.
    p. cm.
    Includes bibliographical references and index.
    ISBN 0-7619-0242-2 (cloth: acid-free paper)
    1. Aged—Institutional care—Evaluation. 2. Old age homes—
Evaluation. 3. Nursing homes—Evaluation. 4. Congregate housing—
Evaluation. 5. Soldier's homes—Evaluation. I. Lemke, Sonne.
II. Title.
HQ1454.M66   1996
362.1'6—dc20   96-9945

96 97 98 99 00 01 02 10 9 8 7 6 5 4 3 2 1

Sage Production Editor: Gillian Dickens
Sage Cover Designer: Candice Harman

Contents

Acknowledgments

Many individuals contributed to this research program, which began more than two decades ago. Jane Clayton, Tom David, Diane Denzler, Mary Gauvain, Joan Kahn, Barbara Mehren, and Eric Postle were responsible for organizing data collection in many of the facilities in the initial sample. A large number of other individuals facilitated the data collection in community residential facilities and in long-term care facilities affiliated with the Department of Veterans Affairs. Bernice Moos helped to organize the data files; she and Diane Denzler, Joan Kahn, Amy Marder, Ann Marten, and Wendy Max conducted the data analyses. The work was supported by NIMH Grant MH28177 and by Department of Veterans Affairs Medical and Health Services Research and Development Service funds. We welcome opportunities to collaborate with or assist others in research or program evaluation in which the MEAP might be a useful tool. We are glad to answer questions and to provide interested investigators with further information about research in progress. If you use the MEAP, we would appreciate learning of your results.

RUDOLF H. MOOS
SONNE LEMKE

1

DEVELOPMENT AND USE OF THE MULTIPHASIC ENVIRONMENTAL ASSESSMENT PROCEDURE

The Multiphasic Environmental Assessment Procedure (MEAP) is a five-part procedure for evaluating the physical and social environments in residential settings for older adults. We designed the procedure to assess nursing homes, residential care facilities, and congregate apartments. The MEAP is designed to be used by qualified clinicians, consultants, program evaluators, and researchers to help them describe and compare facilities, monitor program outcomes, and compare existing facilities with people's preferences.

CONCEPTUAL FRAMEWORK

Development of the MEAP was guided by the conceptual framework presented in Figure 1.1. Panel I of this framework encompasses objective characteristics of the program including the aggregate characteristics of the residents and staff, the physical design of the setting, and the program's policies and services.

Personal factors (Panel II) include the individual resident's socio-demographic characteristics, health, cognitive status, functional ability, and preferences. As indicated by the arrows connecting Panels I and II, the environmental and personal systems influence each other. For exam-

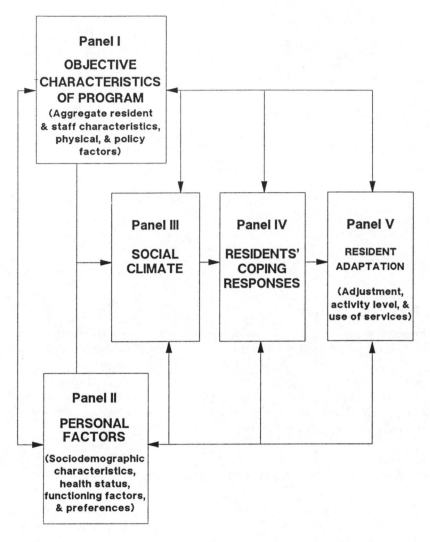

Figure 1.1. A Model of the Relationship Between Program and Personal Factors and Resident Stability and Change

ple, through selection, individuals with particular characteristics (e.g., background and current functioning) are more likely to enter and remain in a given program.

The objective environmental factors and personal factors combine to influence the quality of the program's social climate (Panel III), residents' coping responses (Panel IV), and their adaptation (Panel V). Thus, the model depicts the ongoing interplay between individuals and their residential environments. For example, residents who push for a more active role in facility governance may influence the development of residents' committees and may in turn experience an increased sense of personal efficacy. Such objective changes in the organizational environment and subjective changes in individual self-concept may combine to alter the social climate (e.g., increasing resident influence) and resident outcomes (e.g., improving morale) even for residents who are not directly involved.

This framework applies equally to a variety of residential programs and helps highlight the domains of variables that should be included in comprehensive program evaluation. We developed the MEAP to measure the domains of environmental variables in Panels I and III of the framework; various other instruments are available to measure attributes included in Panels II, IV, and V. Unlike procedures with a narrower focus, the MEAP helps people to describe facilities in an integrated way, understand the differences among facilities, and examine how various facets of the environment interrelate—for example, how architectural features may influence the social climate.

The framework also highlights the fact that a given environmental feature can vary in the way it affects different residents. Congruence theories have been developed to help account for the nature of the interaction between individual residents and a residential environment (e.g., Carp & Carp, 1984; Lawton, 1982, 1989). Currently, we do not have a common metric for measuring persons and environments and therefore cannot specify the presence of person-environment congruence apart from either the subjective appraisal of the individual or the behavioral and affective outcomes of specific combinations of the environmental and individual factors (for a more extended discussion of the framework and of congruence issues, see Moos & Lemke, 1994).

THE MEAP INSTRUMENTS

The MEAP comprises five instruments that measure different aspects of a residential facility. Table 1.1 gives an overview of the instruments,

TABLE 1.1 Overview of the MEAP Instruments

Instrument	Aspect of Environment Assessed	Source
Resident and Staff Information Form (RESIF)	Suprapersonal factors such as the average background and personal characteristics of people living or working in the facility (six subscales)	Records, interviews, and staff reports
Physical and Architectural Features Checklist (PAF)	Physical features including locale, features inside and outside the facility, and space allowances (eight subscales)	Direct observation
Policy and Program Information Form (POLIF)	Facility policies including rules, how the facility is organized, and what services are provided (nine subscales)	Facility administrator and staff reports
Sheltered Care Environment Scale (SCES)	Social milieu including quality of relationships, personal growth emphasis, and system maintenance and change (seven subscales)	Resident and staff reports
Rating Scale	Physical environment and resident and staff functioning (four subscales)	Direct observation

which are used to obtain information about a facility from a number of sources including direct observation, interviews with administrators and other staff, review of facility records, and residents' and staff members' reports of the facility's social climate.

In general, the five instruments correspond with the domains of environmental variables in Figure 1.1. The Resident and Staff Information Form (RESIF) characterizes residents and staff members. The Physical and Architectural Features Checklist (PAF) measures physical features, and the Policy and Program Information Form (POLIF) assesses policies and services. The Sheltered Care Environment Scale (SCES) taps the social climate. The content of the Rating Scale overlaps with that of the other measures; it covers physical features as well as resident and staff characteristics. We kept the Rating Scale separate because it is based on observers' evaluative judgments.

We adapted three of the instruments to measure preferences. The Ideal Forms of the PAF, POLIF, and SCES show what residents, staff, or other respondents would like to see in residences for older adults.

THE BOOK IN BRIEF

This book describes the five MEAP instruments and discusses their use. It replaces the 1992 *MEAP User's Guide* (Moos & Lemke, 1992a) and individual manuals (Moos & Lemke, 1992b, 1992c, 1992d, 1992e, 1992f). Chapter 1 includes an introduction to environmental assessment, a presentation of the ideas behind the MEAP and the sample and methods used to construct it, and a discussion of some practical applications of the MEAP. Chapter 2 contains practical suggestions for administering the MEAP and giving feedback about the results.

We then describe the MEAP's five main parts, which cover the characteristics of the residents and staff in a facility (Chapter 3), a facility's physical features (Chapter 4), its policies and services (Chapter 5), residents' and staff members' appraisals of the facility social climate (Chapter 6), and observers' judgments of a facility's physical features and resident and staff functioning (Chapter 7). Each of these chapters covers the rationale and development of one part of the MEAP, its normative and psychometric characteristics, administration and scoring instructions, and illustrations of how it can be used to describe residential settings for older people. Chapter 8 summarizes some of the findings from research using the MEAP.

CONCEPTUAL BACKGROUND AND DEVELOPMENT

Professionals often have questions about the ideas behind the MEAP and how we constructed and validated the MEAP instruments. Here, we comment on some of the most important issues.

Development of the MEAP

Two major phases of research were involved in developing the MEAP. In the first phase, we used data from group residences in northern California to construct an initial version of the instruments. In the second phase, we used data from a national sample of community facilities to revise the instruments.

Preliminary Version of the MEAP. We identified potential items for the MEAP from several sources including observations in group residences; interviews with residents, staff, and administrators; and discussions with state and local inspectors. We also conducted a thorough search of the literature, reviewed other measurement instruments, and examined published descriptions of residential settings.

We used preliminary versions of the five parts of the MEAP in 93 facilities in northern California. These facilities were located in urban, suburban, and rural settings and varied in type of ownership. The facilities we selected had a minimum of 10 residents and offered at least a meal plan. Considering the level of care and services provided by the facility, we divided the sample into nursing homes, residential care facilities, and congregate apartments. Using these data, as well as conceptual and empirical criteria, we selected items and placed each item on a particular subscale.

Revision of the MEAP. In the second phase, we applied this initial version of the MEAP to 169 community facilities in 20 states. To obtain a varied sample of facilities, we identified urban, suburban, and rural areas in each major geographic region of the United States. Local project assistants helped select suitable facilities, recruited their participation, and collected data. In general, we sampled facilities in the same way as in the California sample. Because the MEAP appeared to be applicable to a broader range of facilities, however, we also included some residential care facilities with fewer than 10 residents and some congregate apartments that did not offer a meal plan.

Scale Construction

We used both conceptual and empirical methods to develop the MEAP subscales. Each item was included in only one subscale so that the subscales would be more distinct. To be included in the MEAP, each item had to

be relevant to the entire range of residential facilities for older people;
have a reasonable response distribution—that is, not be answered the same way in all facilities;
discriminate significantly among facilities;
be conceptually and empirically related to its subscale.

We used these criteria during the two major phases of MEAP development. In the first phase, we used data from facilities in northern California to construct an initial version. In the second phase, we used data from the national sample of community facilities to develop the current version of the MEAP. Chapters 3 through 7 describe the development of each instrument and include the means, standard deviations, internal consistencies, and subscale intercorrelations for each instrument.

Normative Samples

We have normative data for the MEAP from two sets of facilities for older adults: community facilities and facilities serving veterans (for additional information about these samples, see Moos & Lemke, 1994).

Community Facilities. The 262 community facilities include 93 facilities in northern California and 169 facilities in other regions of the United States. These facilities were selected to reflect the variety of residential settings available for elderly adults. Because of similarities in facility characteristics, we combined the California and national samples into a single normative group that includes 135 nursing homes, 60 residential care facilities, and 67 congregate apartments.

The nursing homes provide 24-hour professional nursing care, personal care, and daily living assistance to residents; this sample includes skilled nursing facilities and some homes licensed as intermediate care facilities. On average, the nursing homes have just over 100 residents and a staffing level of 72 full-time staff members for every 100 residents. About two thirds of the nursing homes are proprietary; the remaining one third are nonprofit facilities administered by public agencies or by fraternal or religious groups.

The residential care facilities provide personal care and daily living assistance but not nursing care as standard services to all residents. Among the types of facilities included are personal care sections of continuing care homes and homes licensed as adult group or family homes. Compared with the nursing homes, they are smaller (average size of 80 residents) and provide a lower staffing level (41 staff for every 100 residents, on the average). Almost two thirds of the residential care facilities are proprietary; the remainder are run by nonprofit groups.

Although the congregate apartments generally offer a meal plan, they provide minimal or temporary health, administrative, and personal care services. As a consequence, the staffing level is low (an average of seven

TABLE 1.2 Selected Facility and Resident Characteristics in the Three
Community Subsamples

	Nursing Homes (n = 135 Facilities)		Residential Care (n = 60 Facilities)		Apartments (n = 67 Facilities)	
	Mean	SD	Mean	SD	Mean	SD
Facility characteristics						
Size (number of residents)	104	60	80	84	194	88
Number of staff per 100 residents	72	17	41	19	7	7
% Female staff	88	8	76	23	48	22
% Staff employed more than 1 year	56	23	68	24	63	29
Resident characteristics						
Average age (years)	79	5	79	6	76	4
% Women	69	17	68	25	76	13
% Widowed	61	19	65	22	66	15
% Married	14	10	7	8	15	9
% Divorced	8	8	11	15	11	11
% Never married	17	12	18	17	9	7
% In residence more than 1 year	61	21	71	20	80	24

staff members for every 100 residents). On average, the apartment
facilities house just under 200 residents. This category of facilities
encompasses federally assisted housing for older people, single-room
occupancy hotels, and independent apartments in continuing care facilities. More than 80% of the apartments are nonprofit; the remainder are
proprietary.

Table 1.2 provides summary information on the three sets of facilities
including their size, staffing characteristics, and selected resident background characteristics. Compared with the overall population of persons
over age 60, residents in these congregate living situations are older,
more likely to be women, and more likely to be widowed. Apartment
facilities have the highest proportion of long-term residents and nursing
homes have the lowest. The nursing homes also experience the highest
staff turnover. The facilities providing more services tend to be staffed
by women, whereas those with the fewest services tend to draw equal
numbers of men and women staff.

TABLE 1.3 Selected Facility and Resident Characteristics in the Two Veterans
Subsamples

	Nursing Care Units (N = 57 Facilities)		Domiciliaries (N = 67 Facilities)	
	Mean	SD	Mean	SD
Facility characteristics				
Size (number of residents)	82	83	128	92
Number of staff per 100 residents	84	25	32	15
% Female staff	70	15	55	15
% Staff employed more than 1 year	74	20	85	17
Resident characteristics				
Average age (years)	71	4	68	6
% Women	4	7	12	27
% Widowed	17	10	23	19
% Married	38	12	13	15
% Divorced	18	10	35	19
% Never married	28	12	28	14
% In residence more than 1 year	65	21	74	14

Veterans Facilities. The 81 veterans facilities, like the community sample, were drawn from various regions of the United States. The facilities
include 57 veterans nursing care units and 24 domiciliaries.

The 57 veterans nursing care units include 36 nursing home units and
21 long-term care units. On average, these units house 82 residents and
have a staffing level of 84 full-time staff members for every 100 residents.
These veterans facilities are comparable in their services with the nursing
homes in the community sample.

The 24 domiciliaries include 9 Department of Veterans Affairs-run
domiciliaries and 15 domiciliary sections in state veterans homes. These
units, with an average of 128 residents, are somewhat larger than the
veterans nursing care units and have fewer staff members—on average,
32 staff per 100 residents. Like residential care facilities, they provide
their residents some help with personal care and daily activities, but they
do not provide nursing care to the majority. Half of the veterans facilities
house only men, one serves women and a few married couples, and the
remainder range from 1% to about 30% women.

Table 1.3 summarizes some of the characteristics of these facilities and
their residents. Their largely male population is similar in age distribu-

tion to the population of men over age 60 but unlike them in their marital status—with more in the never-married and divorced categories.

The staffing level is higher in veterans nursing care units than in nursing homes but somewhat lower in domiciliaries than in residential care settings. Compared with community facilities, more of the staff in veterans facilities have worked there more than a year and more of them are men.

Measuring the Overall Quality
of a Facility

We have combined subscales from the MEAP instruments into eight indices of quality. These quality indices, which cover the physical setting, policies and services, and social climate, can be applied to all three levels of care. We formulated preliminary indices by agreement among three judges and then revised them on the basis of their variability (both between and within levels of care), their internal coherence, and their independence of each other. (For more information on these indices, see Lemke & Moos, 1986.)

The first four indices reflect the structure of care:

1. Staff Resources is the RESIF subscale that measures the resources available from staff in terms of their experience, diversity, and training.
2. Staffing level is the ratio of full-time equivalent staff members to residents.
3. Comfort measures how spacious and pleasant the physical setting is by averaging the facility score on three of the PAF subscales—Physical Amenities, Social-Recreational Aids, and Space Availability.
4. Security measures the presence of physical features that support optimum functioning. This index is the average of the facility scores on the PAF subscales of Prosthetic Aids, Orientational Aids, and Safety Features.

The remaining four indices focus on the process of care:

5. Autonomy is the average of scores on the POLIF subscales of Policy Choice, Resident Control, and Provision for Privacy.
6. Services combines POLIF subscales that measure the provision of three types of services: health care, daily living assistance, and social-recreational activities.
7. Rapport reflects residents' perceptions concerning the warmth, freedom from conflict, supportiveness, and smooth functioning of relationships among

residents and between staff and residents. The index combines scores on the SCES Cohesion, Conflict (reversed), and Organization subscales.

8. Control measures residents' perceptions of how independent and influential they are in the facility. This index combines scores on the SCES Independence and Resident Influence subscales.

Measuring People's Preferences About Residential Facilities

After developing the basic MEAP instruments, we constructed Ideal Forms as a parallel method to tap preferences about design and program characteristics. We have had residents, staff, and older adults who live in their own homes complete the Ideal Forms. Other individuals, such as family members of residents, can also complete them. Professionals can use the results to compare the preferences of different groups, to examine individual variations in preferences, and to measure person-environment congruence. (For more information about potential applications, see Brennan, Moos, & Lemke, 1988, 1989; Moos, Lemke, & David, 1987).

We reworded PAF, POLIF, and SCES items to elicit information about preferences. For example, the PAF item "Are there handrails in the halls?" became "Should there be handrails in the halls?" We phrased items as questions so they could be administered as a written inventory or in an interview. After a series of trials and revisions, we constructed the PAF Form I, which includes seven of the eight PAF subscales, and the POLIF Form I, which has all nine POLIF subscales.

We administered the PAF Form I and POLIF Form I to nine groups of respondents including residents and staff from nursing homes, residential care facilities, and congregate apartments; current residents of an apartment asked to respond in terms of a new nursing home; community residents asked to rate an ideal congregate apartment; and gerontologists who conduct research and evaluate residential settings for older people. (For more normative and psychometric information, see Chapters 3 and 4, this volume; Brennan et al., 1988, 1989.)

We developed the SCES Form I to parallel the SCES Form R. Form I asks people how they conceive of the social climate of an ideal group residence. Because the two forms have a parallel set of 63 items, the SCES facilitates comparisons of actual and preferred environments and of resident and staff preferences. (For preliminary normative and psychometric data for SCES Form I, see Chapter 5.)

The Validity of the MEAP

We built content and face validity into the MEAP from the outset by

defining constructs such as community accessibility, policy clarity, and cohesion;

preparing items to fit the construct definitions;

grouping items that are conceptually related into subscales;

evaluating these conceptual groupings according to empirical criteria such as item intercorrelations and item-subscale correlations.

In addition, the MEAP instruments show evidence of construct validity—that is, subscales tend to differentiate between types of facilities and interrelate in expected ways. There are strong associations between MEAP subscales that assess conceptually similar dimensions from the perspective of different groups of observers. For example, several of the PAF subscales are positively related to the quality of the physical environment as reported by observers using the Rating Scale. Moreover, residents report greater comfort in facilities that provide more physical amenities, social-recreational aids, and space, as well as in facilities that observers rate higher on physical attractiveness and environmental diversity (Moos & Lemke, 1994). Information obtained from the administrator about how much residents are involved in running the facility (POLIF Resident Control) is highly related to the residents' perceptions of the amount of influence they have (SCES Resident Influence).

In general, the findings identify expected relationships among the MEAP subscales and provide evidence of their construct validity. (For an extended discussion of some aspects of the construct validity of the SCES, see Lemke & Moos, 1990; Smith & Whitbourne, 1990.)

Criterion validity of the MEAP is acceptable; the dimensions are related to external criteria in both concurrent and predictive studies. For example, resident and staff perceptions of the social climate are predictably related to social workers' ratings of nursing home quality (Stein, Linn, & Stein, 1987). We found that in facilities that have a high level of resident control and that establish a cohesive and resident-directed social climate, residents are more likely to participate in self-initiated activities in the facility and in the community. In programs that are more structured and well staffed, residents are more likely to participate in activities sponsored by the facility (Lemke & Moos, 1989b).

Overall, the findings indicate that the MEAP subscales show reasonably good construct and criterion validity. The subsequent chapters address issues of validity in more detail (also see Moos & Lemke, 1994).

APPLICATIONS FOR PRACTITIONERS
AND PROGRAM EVALUATORS

The MEAP can help practitioners and program evaluators understand the basic dimensions of residential settings, how they influence people, and how people adapt to them. These insights can improve consultation and program interventions.

The MEAP gives residents and staff a new framework for thinking about their facility. Instead of viewing it in terms of high or low quality, they can see it as multidimensional. The MEAP helps people view the setting as a whole and consider its impact on all residents. This approach encourages flexibility by pointing out different avenues for carrying out change.

Using the MEAP and giving feedback can raise important issues—for example, regarding the nature of administrator and staff roles, the clarity of and consensus about facility policies, and sources of resistance to change. When staff members discuss these issues openly, they are more motivated to try to improve their facility and better able to successfully carry out planned changes.

The MEAP can also help students and professionals to understand residential facilities. Students of social gerontology have used the SCES to describe facilities and compare their own reports with those of residents and staff; this exercise helps students to think about the important aspects of the social climate and their potential impact (Waters, 1981). In addition, social workers, community volunteers, residents' family members, and others can use the MEAP instruments, especially the Rating Scale and SCES, to report their impressions of a facility.

Descriptive information indicating how typical or unique a facility is can also help indicate whether an intervention is likely to generalize to other facilities. For example, prior to a manipulation to increase personal control in a nursing home, Johnson (1981) used the POLIF to show that the home was comparable to the normative sample in the level of institutional constraint; the results she obtained are therefore likely to generalize to other nursing facilities.

Evaluating Program Implementation

To determine how well a program is implemented, the actual program must be compared against a standard of what the program should be. To focus on this issue, we have used three sources of information to define a standard for program implementation: normative data on conditions in other programs, which allow an evaluator to see how one program compares with others; specification of an ideal program; and conceptual analysis or expert judgment.

Normative Standards. MEAP results can be used to portray a facility and to evaluate program implementation by comparison with normative standards. One of the most useful approaches is to profile the results as standard scores (with a mean of 50 and a standard deviation of 10) based on the appropriate normative sample. The resulting profiles identify areas in which the facility has more or fewer resources than other facilities offering a similar level of care.

By depicting the results visually, MEAP profiles help to develop detailed descriptions of residential facilities. Chapters 3 through 7 illustrate some of these applications by presenting profiles of a community nursing home, a residential care facility, and a congregate apartment. (For additional examples of MEAP profiles, see Moos & Lemke, 1994; Moos et al., 1987; Timko & Moos, 1991a).

Thompson and Swisher (1983) used portions of the MEAP in this manner to describe the apartment section of a new, continuing-care facility. The facility was average or above average on most physical features, especially safety features and space; it also gave residents privacy, choice in activities of daily living, and opportunities for participation in facility governance. Consistent with these findings, the residents saw the facility as cohesive, well organized, oriented toward self-direction, and comfortable. In contrast, the staff reported only average emphasis in most areas; physical comfort was well below average. Thus, the SCES identified differences between residents' and staff's views of how well this new program was being implemented.

Specification of an Ideal Program. For another perspective on program implementation, program evaluators can use Form I of the PAF, POLIF, or SCES, which gives respondents the opportunity to describe their ideal residential facility. Comparison of Form R and Form I of the MEAP instruments reflects how well the current program matches the preferred program as illustrated in Chapters 4, 5, and 6. Such comparisons provide a more complete picture of the implementation of a program and better insight into problem areas. For example, Waters (1980a) administered Form R and Form I of the SCES to staff in a private long-term care facility. The differences between the real and ideal scores indicated that the staff wanted more emphasis on cohesion, independence, organization, and physical comfort and less on conflict (see also Waters, 1980b).

Information from the Ideal Form can also be used to make individual-level comparisons between a person's preferences and the characteristics of an actual facility (e.g., see Moos et al., 1987). A group-level comparison can be made by determining whether a facility provides the specific characteristics that are rated very important or essential by a specific proportion (such as 25%) of its residents or of a group of potential residents.

The Ideal Forms can also provide information on how much people agree with each other about their preferred facility. For example, program evaluators can compare the physical features that administrators and staff value, the policies that current residents and those on a waiting list want, or the amount of independence that nursing home and congregate apartment residents prefer.

Conceptual Analysis and Expert Judgment. Blake (1985-1986, 1987) used descriptive information about group homes for frail elderly and mentally ill residents to evaluate whether they achieve their intended goal of providing a noninstitutional therapeutic environment. The group homes he evaluated had relatively restrictive policies and offered few health services or activities. He concluded that the programs were not well implemented in that they did not provide a normal living situation nor were they oriented toward rehabilitation.

In a similar approach, Mowbray, Greenfield, and Freddolino (1992) assessed the adequacy and appropriateness of the program offered by small group homes. They found that these homes required independence in self-care and an absence of problem behaviors from their residents and that residents rarely participated in decision making. They concluded that these homes serve clients who are capable of living in more independent settings and exclude clients for whom their services would be appropriate. In addition, although they offer a home-like environment in some respects, they have a number of institutional qualities (lack of variation and of personalization of the physical environment and top-down decision making).

Chambers and colleagues (1988) specified a program standard by describing the principles underlying a community mental health promotion program for residential facilities. They then used the MEAP to help develop guidelines to evaluate how well specific therapeutic environments conformed to these principles.

Monitoring Interventions

The MEAP can indicate whether an intervention program is having the intended consequences. Studies formulated along these lines have examined program enrichment and relocation. (For an example of the use of the SCES to monitor changes in social climate associated with a change in facility ownership, see Chapter 6.)

Program Enrichment. Berkowitz, Waxman, and Yaffe (1988) used the SCES to evaluate the influence of an enriched self-help program on resident well-being and on the social climate of a congregate apartment building. New, professionally trained staff were added to the target housing unit, and residents were encouraged to participate in decision making; two other apartment buildings were comparison sites. As predicted, residents in the self-help housing model reported more cohesion, independence, and resident influence as well as higher self-esteem. In this example, the SCES showed that the new program was well implemented as indexed by residents' perceptions.

Following a special training program for nursing home staff, Spinner (1986/1985) used the SCES to evaluate its impact on the social climate of the nursing home. Staff in the homes with the training program reported higher self-disclosure and resident influence than did staff in the control homes; residents' scores did not differentiate between the treatment and control homes. Staff training may improve the work climate of nursing homes, but more intensive and long-term training may be needed to show an impact on the social climate experienced by residents.

Byerts and Heller (1985) used several parts of the MEAP to compare a service-enhanced congregate housing facility with five regular housing sites. As expected, the enhanced facility actually had more health and daily living services, indicating that key aspects of the program had been successfully implemented. The enhanced and regular sites were comparable in physical features and in resident and staff composition, but residents in the enhanced site had fewer social resources and were less likely to participate in activities.

These differences in selection of residents, as well as failure to meet all of the residents' heightened expectations, may explain why seniors who moved into the service-enhanced housing reported poorer personal adjustment and less satisfaction with housing quality and services received despite their lower mortality rate at a 3-year follow-up. In this case, the MEAP helped to show that the program may have had some undesired impacts.

Relocation. In relocation studies, the MEAP can document the overall quality of the settings and the similarity between the old and new environments. Such information can be shared with administrators and staff and can be used to clarify the new environmental challenges residents and staff face and to help maximize the positive impact of relocation.

In one study of an intrainstitutional relocation, for example, the PAF showed that the existing facility offered a variety of social-recreational aids, a relatively spacious physical environment, and easy orientation but lacked the prosthetic and safety features often valued by older people. The new facility provided a richer physical environment with more prosthetic aids, but the building was also larger and more complex. In addition, communal social spaces were located some distance from staff caregiving areas. Residents changed their behavior in predictable ways to try to adapt to the larger design and altered layout of the new facility (Moos, David, Lemke, & Postle, 1984).

Planning and Improving Facilities

The MEAP is a valuable resource in designing new programs and in improving established ones. The MEAP can help administrators and staff understand the dynamics of their setting, clarify their goals, suggest ways to improve the facility, and assess the results of a program of change.

The process of systematically improving a facility has four steps: (a) assessing the environment, (b) giving feedback on the results of the assessment, (c) planning and instituting change, and (d) reassessing the environment. (For examples, see Finney & Moos, 1984; Moos, 1988a; Moos & Lemke, 1983.) Several projects illustrate this process.

Organizational Development in Nursing Homes. Wells (1990) has described an empowerment model for engaging planners, service providers, residents, and families of residents in a collaborative process to improve the quality of life in long-term care facilities. Wells and colleagues conducted a 3-year demonstration project using a matched-pair comparison group design in four skilled nursing facilities (see also Wells, 1990; Wells & Singer, 1988; Wells, Singer, & Polgar, 1986).

Initial findings identified problems such as policies that allowed residents little choice or involvement in facility planning and buildings that lacked orientational aids. After the findings were presented to staff, committees made up of residents, staff, and family members were organized to identify the most important problem areas and make changes. These committees planned such changes as an increase in orientational aids, a subcommittee to welcome new residents and their families, an information brochure for new residents, and a self-help group to increase residents' confidence in public speaking.

Overall, the change process improved residents' attitudes, promoted awareness of quality of life issues, and led to changes in organizational procedures and to better communication among various groups. Residents formed closer relationships, communicated more openly with each other, became more confident and skillful in presenting their ideas, and began to take a much more active role in facility governance. They reported gains in self-esteem, sense of affiliation, and satisfaction. Moreover, nursing audits showed that residents who participated in the resident groups needed less nursing care.

The MEAP and feedback from it fostered the organizational development project in four main ways: (a) as a model of the way the project should work; (b) as a catalyst for discussion; (c) as a means of helping the social worker develop task-oriented contacts with residents, staff, and families; and (d) as a focus for identifying areas in which to initiate change.

Improving the Quality of Group Homes. Hatcher, Gentry, Kunkel, and Smith (1983) conducted a project to improve the quality of life of residents in group homes. They used the MEAP to identify targets for change and to document the actual changes made. In one home, community workers collaborated with the manager and residents to establish a residents' council, plan activities in the community, and add some orientational aids. As expected, policy choice, resident activities in the community, and orientational aids increased. In another home, the intervention was designed to raise the manager's expectations for resident functioning and to increase involvement in facility-provided and self-initiated activities. In general, these goals were achieved; the level of resident choice and control in the home also increased. In this project, the MEAP provided community workers with a concrete method for setting change goals and evaluating progress made in meeting them.

Improving the Quality of Congregate Apartments. Fernandez-Ballesteros and colleagues (Fernandez-Ballesteros, Diaz, Izal, & Gonzalez, 1986; Fernandez-Ballesteros et al., 1987) used a Spanish version of the MEAP to assess a large congregate apartment facility. The findings highlighted the need to increase prosthetic and orientational aids, facilitate social interaction, and promote resident participation and independence. Accordingly, the staff made some changes in the physical environment (such as having an entrance ramp constructed, creating new recreational areas, and rearranging furniture) and facility policies (such as allowing the residents to use the bulletin boards for announcements).

The changes led to increased resident participation in facility-sponsored and community activities as well as to a greater sense of independence and influence on the residents' part. After the changes were made, the residents also reported more conflict, and the staff appraised the facility as less comfortable; these findings may reflect the residents' enhanced activity and self-confidence and staff's negative reaction to the development of a more resident-oriented environment. More generally, the findings highlight the value of a comprehensive assessment to identify the unintended effects of program changes.

Enhancing Problem Solving and Facility Design. Aside from using the MEAP to identify targets for change and to document the impact of change efforts, the MEAP can be adapted in other ways to facilitate program improvement. Parts of the MEAP can be used as a checklist during the planning of a new facility. Designers and planners can consider both what future residents want and how physical design and program factors may affect residents.

In an existing facility, evaluators can observe how residents adapt to the facility and can identify ways to improve it. In such an application, Deutschman (1982) asked staff to use an adapted version of the PAF to identify key problems in their environment. After reviewing the information, a team of architects, interior designers, and health care practitioners developed a handbook to provide staff with a range of innovative, low-cost solutions for the most frequent architectural problems in long-term care facilities.

RESEARCH APPLICATIONS

Paralleling these practical applications, the MEAP has a variety of research uses. These research applications examine the panels and processes depicted in Figure 1.1. At the most basic level, researchers can use the MEAP to describe the residential settings under study.

A second research goal is to try to understand the patterns of relationships among environmental attributes. For example, how are resident characteristics related to the physical resources available in the facility, to the policies and organizational structure that develop, or to the facility's social climate? By expanding the scope somewhat, researcher, can investigate how facility characteristics, such as ownership or size, relate to the resources available to residents and staff. Developing program typologies, which capture the patterns of co-occurrence among MEAP dimensions, can help reduce the amount of discrete information that must be considered.

In addition to looking at the precursors of a facility's features and resources, researchers can examine their consequences for staff and residents both at the group and at the individual levels. Here, researchers are concerned with whether some programs are more effective than others and, if so, what features contribute to their effectiveness. As with all program outcome research, these rather straightforward questions about outcomes quickly multiply into questions about differential impact on various outcomes (e.g., an intervention may improve morale but reduce residents' activity levels) and differential impact on various groups (e.g., a prosthetic feature may improve mobility for some subgroups of residents but not for others). We summarize findings from research that has addressed these issues in Chapter 8.

2

ADMINISTRATION, SCORING, AND GIVING FEEDBACK

Before you use the Multiphasic Environmental Assessment Procedure (MEAP) to characterize a residential setting, you will need to make arrangements for data collection and set project guidelines. In this chapter, we give some suggestions for handling these and other practical issues.

Encouraging Cooperation

Because many people must cooperate in the completion of the MEAP, you must take particular care in presenting it, setting up procedures for its administration, and setting guidelines about confidentiality and about reporting results. To encourage cooperation, point out the unique nature of the information that can be obtained. Decide ahead of time whether you will give feedback on the MEAP results; if you plan to do so, emphasize this benefit of participation.

Administrators have various reasons for being cautious about having their facilities evaluated with the MEAP. The following are examples of possible concerns that administrators may have as well as suggestions for handling each concern:

1. If the administrator is afraid that the "negative" nature of some questions may make the facility look bad, explain that residents and staff

can answer "no" to these questions and that to assess the variety of facilities available, such questions need to be included. This reservation may also reflect a concern that negative results will be disseminated to the press or to advocacy groups. You should therefore be explicit about how results will be used and who will be allowed to share them.

2. If the administrator is concerned that the MEAP will reflect a temporary condition in the facility, such as a change of organization or administration, you should acknowledge that possibility. You may wish to offer to do a follow-up after conditions have stabilized.

3. If the administrator wonders how some staff ("troublemakers") or residents ("complainers" or confused or suspicious residents) may affect the Sheltered Care Environment Scale (SCES) results, explain that the SCES profile reflects the impressions of all the staff or residents who complete the questionnaire. The responses of a few dissenters will be averaged into the whole and will usually have a minimal effect on the profile. In addition, confused or very suspicious residents usually either cannot or will not complete the questionnaire.

4. Particularly in nursing homes, the administrator may express the fear that completing questionnaires may upset the residents. Note that in most cases the process is positive for older residents, who enjoy talking to someone interested in their views about the facility. In addition, assure the administrator that you will not pressure residents to participate and that you will explain to all potential respondents that their participation is voluntary.

5. If the administrator warns that residents or staff will refuse to participate for some reason (e.g., apathetic, too busy, unionized, or a bad experience with research in the past), ask the administrator for suggestions about how to approach the staff and residents to maximize participation.

Initial Meeting With the Facility Administrator

In your first meeting with the facility administrator, review the instruments that you want to use. Ask the administrator about the best sources of information for the Policy and Program Information Form (POLIF) and Resident and Staff Information Form (RESIF)—that is, should you obtain data from records, a particular staff member, or residents? Discuss ways to maximize the return rate on the SCES when you administer it to residents and staff.

Use this information to outline a proposed timetable for data collection, and review your proposal with the administrator; then use the timetable to schedule appointments and request records in advance. Try to minimize interference with the facility's other activities. If the administrator will not give you access to records, ask if you can pay a facility employee to tabulate these data.

After you obtain the administrator's permission to study the facility, meet with residents and staff to describe the SCES and to ask for their support. The personal contact usually results in a higher participation rate. Chapter 6 discusses some additional procedures for administering the SCES and giving feedback.

Setting Policies About Confidentiality and the Use of MEAP Results

Most people see the physical and social characteristics of settings as important; people usually are interested in helping with the assessment and want to learn more about these characteristics and their effects. Facility administrators, other staff, and residents, however, will want to know how you plan to use the MEAP results. Usually, they will be concerned with questions of anonymity, confidentiality, and sharing of overall results. You should raise and discuss these questions early on. Your decisions will depend on circumstances that vary from project to project including the purpose of the study, whether you are a staff member of the facility that you are studying, and how you recruited facilities to participate in the study.

In handling these questions, try to adhere to the following general guidelines. First, when administering the SCES, gather data anonymously if possible. If you need to connect individual responses to other individual measures, such as comparing SCES scores with measures of self-confidence, then use coding to ensure anonymity. Second, keep individual results confidential. Finally, give overall results to the people in the facility before giving them to others; you might offer to show the participants how their facility compares with other similar facilities or how the facility changes over time.

Defining the Unit

In cases of self-contained, homogeneous living environments, the unit of study will be easy to define. When the facility offers several levels of care or has a number of discrete units, carefully think through how to define the unit of study and how this decision affects specific sections of the MEAP. When questions arise, be guided by functional considerations. For example, what do residents and staff define as the living units of the facility? Sections offering different levels of care should generally be treated as separate units.

Consider actual availability and use when you define access to staff, services, and physical resources for each unit. For example, in the case of a congregate apartment that is attached to a nursing home, certain nursing home services, programs, and physical spaces can be counted as available to apartment residents as long as the individual is not required to move to the nursing home to use them. Thus, an apartment resident may be able to receive physical therapy in the nursing home during specific hours, and this should be indicated on the POLIF.

As another example, a recreation hall may be available to a number of units within a complex. Only those units whose residents actually use the recreation hall should be counted as having access to it even though there may be no prohibition against all residents using it. That is, if residents in a nursing home have their activities within the nursing home rather than in a recreation hall, the nursing home should not be credited with resources in the recreation hall.

Define the unit under study before beginning the data collection; this will help you avoid inefficiency or duplication of effort. You can collect information from subunits of a facility and then combine them into a single unit where appropriate.

Selecting MEAP Instruments

We view a residential facility as a dynamic system that includes aggregate resident and staff characteristics, physical features, policies and services, and social climate. The MEAP creates an integrated picture of a facility by using various sources of information to describe these domains. We designed the MEAP so that the instruments can be used individually or in any combination. Using them in combination creates a more complete picture of a residential facility because it uses more sources of information, shows how physical and social factors interact, and helps you anticipate how changes in one area may affect other areas.

The purpose of your clinical or research work will determine the particular instruments you should use. For example, if you are primarily interested in the policies and services in the facility, the POLIF will provide the relevant information. If you want to know more about how residents and staff perceive a facility, use the SCES. The following are guidelines on the time required to complete each instrument:

Two hours may be required for an experienced data collector to complete the Physical and Architectural Features Checklist (PAF)—schedule more time if the facility is large or complex.

One hour may be required to complete the POLIF if the administrator is knowledgeable and the information is accessible and well organized.

Three hours may be required to locate and tabulate RESIF data in a facility with 100 residents.

About 30 minutes may be required to administer the SCES to a group; the SCES can also be self-administered. If you need to read the items to residents, as is the case in most nursing homes, plan to spend from 15 to 30 minutes with each resident.

Only a few extra minutes should be required for the Rating Scale if you complete it while filling out the PAF.

Administering the Ideal Forms

Each MEAP instrument describes a facility as it is. In addition, the PAF, POLIF, and SCES each has a corresponding Form I (Ideal Form) for describing a preferred or an ideal facility.

The purpose of your work will determine whether you want to use the Ideal Forms. For example, a comparison between a facility's PAF results and PAF Form I results provides important information about respondents' preferences and suggests areas in which change may be desired.

If you wish to administer both the actual (Form R) and the ideal (Form I) forms of the SCES, administer each form in a different session. This reduces fatigue and helps people keep their impressions of their current environment separate from their ideas about a preferred setting. Similarly, if you wish to administer Form I of the PAF and the POLIF, do so in separate sessions to reduce fatigue.

People usually need 15 to 30 minutes to complete the SCES Form I, 1 hour to complete the PAF Form I, and 1 hour to complete the POLIF Form I.

Options for Administering
Questionnaires to Residents and Staff

Practically achievable response rates for questionnaires from residents vary considerably among facilities. In most cases, over 60% of residents in residential care facilities, domiciliaries, or apartment buildings can complete the SCES or the Ideal Form of the PAF or POLIF. In nursing homes, only 10% to 30% of the residents will be able to complete these questionnaires and only intellectually intact residents should be asked to do so. Because most staff members can complete these questionnaires, achieving high response rates from staff is largely a question of motivating them.

Facility With Many Impaired Residents. Completing the SCES, PAF-I, or POLIF-I is time-consuming in facilities with many impaired residents. To make your work easier, ask the administrator to arrange for the head nurse, the activity director, or another staff member who knows the residents well to prepare a list of residents able to participate. Request that the list include the room number of each of these residents and whether assistance will be needed.

Allow about 30 minutes per resident for administration of the SCES by interview and 1 hour per resident for the PAF-I or the POLIF-I. In addition, allow extra time to assist as needed those residents who are assumed to be able to fill out the questionnaire on their own. Keep in mind that showers, meals, naps, and other activities may interfere with your administration schedule.

When you arrive to administer the questionnaire, find the residents whose names are on the list. If some of these residents are in a communal area, ask a staff member to introduce you to them. Whether you are talking to residents in a group or individually, tell them briefly about the study and the questionnaire; also explain that you have the administrator's permission to ask these questions and that participation is voluntary. Determine which residents need help in reading the questionnaire, marking answers, or both. For residents who can complete the questionnaire independently, arrange to pick up the completed questionnaire later that day.

Facility With High-Functioning Residents. If a facility with high-functioning residents has a tenants' association or other regularly scheduled residents' meeting, you may be able to use this meeting to describe and distribute the questionnaire. To increase attendance at the meeting, place an announcement on the bulletin board or send a letter to residents in which you describe the project and its importance.

At the meeting, ask a staff member to introduce you to the group. Briefly describe the study, the questionnaire, and the residents' role in completing it. Note that their participation is voluntary. Encourage them to complete the questionnaire during or immediately after the meeting but explain that they may complete it in the next day or two if they prefer. Be prepared to provide pencils. Arrange for someone to help residents who need assistance in reading or recording their answers; the collaboration should take place where others will not be disturbed. You can collect completed questionnaires in person, using stamped return envelopes, and via a box in the lobby.

In a facility without community or group meetings, you can send the questionnaire to each resident or, in a large facility, to a sample. Include a cover letter in which you describe the project and note that it has the administrator's approval and that residents' participation is voluntary. Explain when and where participants can get assistance. You can distribute the questionnaire by mail or in person and collect the completed questionnaires in person, using stamped return envelopes, or via a box in the lobby. Distributing questionnaires, assisting residents, and collecting completed questionnaires can take as much as an entire day.

Directions for Having Staff Complete and Return Questionnaires. You can present the SCES, PAF-I, or POLIF-I to staff at a regularly scheduled staff meeting or at a special meeting called for this purpose. Ordinarily, 30 minutes is enough time to describe the study and administer the SCES and 1 hour is enough time to administer the PAF-I or POLIF-I. If the administrator incorporates the evaluation into in-service training, however, you may be asked to describe the project in more detail. Furthermore, in some facilities, reaching all staff may entail scheduling more than one meeting.

Ask the administrator or a supervisor to introduce you to the group. Briefly describe the project and the questionnaire; let staff know that their participation is voluntary. Ask them to complete and return the questionnaire during the meeting. If some staff need to complete and return the questionnaire later, give them stamped, addressed envelopes.

The usual requirements for questionnaire administration apply. Use a quiet, well-lighted room with ample space for each person to work. For less sophisticated respondents, keep the group small enough so that you can circulate around the room and help them as necessary. Be prepared to provide pencils. On request, give simple clarifications of word meanings, but be careful not to influence the direction of the person's response. Encourage respondents to answer each item.

SCORING AND FEEDBACK GUIDELINES

Instructions for scoring the MEAP are included in Appendix B. The raw scores reflect the percentage of items or possible points with which the facility is credited. In contrast, standard scores incorporate information about a facility's characteristics relative to others and allow you to make direct comparisons among subscales. You can easily convert subscale percentage scores to standard scores, which have a mean of 50 and a standard deviation of 10, by using the tables in Appendix C.

Giving Feedback

Giving feedback on the results of the MEAP is as important as obtaining and analyzing the data. You might want to provide information on

> how the MEAP describes the physical features, policies, and services in the setting and how the facility compares with other such settings;
> how different groups compare—for example, how staff and residents see the social climate in the facility;
> how the facility compares with staff and resident preferences.

The exact procedures for giving feedback will depend on the arrangements you make with the facility administrator. Usually, the initial feedback session is open to other people, such as staff members, although sometimes the person in charge wants to see the results first in a private session. Only after the person in charge has reviewed the results and agreed to share them should you relay the information to an administrator at the next higher or lower level. Usually, people want to learn more about their environment. They find the feedback useful and often want to use it to improve the setting.

3

THE RESIDENT AND STAFF
INFORMATION FORM

The Resident and Staff Information Form (RESIF) measures those aspects of a facility that derive from the characteristics of its residents and staff. When individuals come together in a social group, such as a college dormitory, a work group, or a congregate residence for older people, they bring with them abilities, values, and behavioral preferences. Because of selective mechanisms, groups draw their members in a non-random manner from the general population and, in doing so, produce distinctive combinations of these individual characteristics. The aggregate of the members' attributes (the suprapersonal environment) in part defines the subculture that develops in a group, and this subculture in turn can influence the behavior of individual members.

The RESIF is composed of 104 scored items that describe residents and staff in group residences for older people. Information is obtained from interviews with administrators and other staff, observation of residents and staff, review of facility records, and sometimes questionnaires given to residents.

RESIF SUBSCALES

The six RESIF subscales are presented in Table 3.1; they fall into three groups. The first two subscales measure residents' background characteristics. The Resident Social Resources subscale assesses four socio-demographic variables related to social competence. The theory is that

TABLE 3.1 Resident and Staff Information Form (RESIF) Subscale
              Descriptions

Subscale	Description
	Residents' background characteristics
Resident Social Resources	The current status of residents with respect to demographic variables that facilitate social competence
Resident Heterogeneity	The extent to which residents are a diverse group of individuals
	Residents' functioning and activity involvement
Functional Abilities	Residents' independence in performing daily functions and freedom from functional handicaps
Activity Level	The extent to which residents are involved in activities in the facility that they can initiate
Activities in the Community	The rate of residents' participation in activities that take them outside the facility
	Staff characteristics
Staff Resources	The resources available from the staff in terms of experience, training, and variety of backgrounds

residents who have at least some high school education, who had higher-status jobs, who are married, and who do not receive public assistance have more social resources than do their counterparts who lack these attributes. The Resident Heterogeneity subscale measures the diversity of residents with respect to such sociodemographic factors as gender, age, ethnicity, education, and religion.

The next three dimensions tap the residents' current functioning and activity involvement. The Functional Abilities subscale assesses the residents' capacity to perform such daily functions as taking care of their own appearance, eating meals, dressing, and walking. The Activity Level subscale focuses on residents' involvement in activities in the facility that residents can initiate such as listening to music, knitting, engaging in a hobby, and visiting with other residents. The Activities in the Community subscale evaluates residents' participation in activities outside the facility such as visiting friends or relatives, going on a tour, attending religious services, going shopping, and eating out.

The Staff Resources subscale reflects staff members' experience, training, and diversity. Staff Resources is positively related to the staff-resident ratio but taps more varied aspects of the staff resources available to residents. For example, the items include the proportion of staff who have worked in the facility for more than a year, the availability of older staff members, the number of hours volunteers spend in the facility, and the type of in-service training programs for staff.

NORMATIVE SAMPLES AND PSYCHOMETRIC CHARACTERISTICS

Normative Samples

Normative data for the RESIF are available for the two samples of facilities for older adults: the 262 community facilities and the 81 facilities serving veterans (see Normative Samples in Chapter 1).

Items on two of the RESIF subscales (Resident Heterogeneity and Staff Resources) are scored dichotomously. Scoring of some of these items requires transformation of frequencies or percentages into dichotomous distributions. The cutoff points for these items were established on the basis of conceptual criteria and the actual distribution obtained for our sample of facilities. Items on the remaining four subscales are scored in terms of the proportion of residents who have a particular background characteristic or who participate in a specified activity.

Subscale scores are expressed as percentage scores reflecting the sum of item scores in relation to the total points possible. For example, the Activity Level subscale is composed of 13 items, each with a range from 0% to 100%; facility scores can vary from 0% (none of the residents are involved in any of the activities) to 100% (all of the residents are involved in every activity). In a facility that obtains a percentage score of 40%, the average resident is involved in 40% of the activities; looked at another way, on average, 40% of the residents participate in these activities. Hand-scoring worksheets are provided in Appendix B; the standard score conversion table is in Appendix C.

Community Facilities

Means and standard deviations for the six RESIF subscales for the total community sample and for each of the three subsamples are reported in Table 3.2. The sample of community facilities varies considerably on all

TABLE 3.2   RESIF Subscale Means and Standard Deviations for the Total
Community Sample and the Three Subsamples

Subscale	Total Sample (n = 262 Facilities)		Nursing Homes (n = 135 Facilities)		Residential Care (n = 60 Facilities)		Apartments (n = 67 Facilities)	
	Mean	SD	Mean	SD	Mean	SD	Mean	SD
Resident Social Resources[a]	38	17	32	15	46	19	46	15
Resident Heterogeneity	40	21	42	20	34	21	42	24
Functional Abilities	61	27	37	13	78	15	92	5
Activity Level	35	15	26	11	42	12	50	11
Activities in the Community	25	19	15	13	28	16	43	18
Staff Resources	47	20	59	15	40	19	31	15

a. $n = 162$ facilities: 88 nursing homes, 31 residential care facilities, and 43 apartments.

six subscales as shown by the standard deviations in Table 3.2. In general,
the six RESIF subscales discriminate among and between the three types
of facilities, although some of the subscales show less variability among
nursing homes or among apartment facilities.

The three facility types differ somewhat in the demographic characteristics of their residents. On average, residents in nursing homes have
fewer social resources compared with those in residential care and
apartment facilities.

Striking differences between facility types are apparent for the next
three subscales. Functional Abilities, Activity Level, and Activities in the
Community are lowest in nursing homes, intermediate in residential care
facilities, and highest in apartments. Residents in apartments show little
variability on the Functional Abilities subscale because almost all residents can function independently in tasks of daily living. On the other
hand, apartment residents vary considerably on Activity Level and Activities in the Community. Thus, these three subscales can be used
together to tap aspects of functioning and activity involvement of residents in each type of facility.

The staff-resident ratio varies considerably among the three types of
community facilities with little overlap in their distributions. In contrast,

TABLE 3.3 RESIF Subscale Means and Standard Deviations for the Total Veterans Sample and the Two Subsamples

Subscale	Total Sample (n = 81 Facilities)		Nursing Care Units (n = 57 Facilities)		Domiciliaries (n = 24 Facilities)	
	Mean	SD	Mean	SD	Mean	SD
Resident Social Resources[a]	51	8	54	7	44	7
Resident Heterogeneity	40	16	42	14	36	21
Functional Abilities	58	24	44	15	88	9
Activity Level	33	14	28	11	47	11
Activities in the Community	27	17	22	14	39	19
Staff Resources	69	12	70	11	67	14

a. *n* = 73 facilities: 54 nursing care units and 19 domiciliaries.

although Staff Resources is highest in nursing homes and lowest in apartments, there is overlap in the distribution for the three subsamples.

Veterans Facilities

The RESIF means and standard deviations for the sample of 81 veterans facilities and for each of the two subsamples are given in Table 3.3. The veterans in the nursing care units are quite different from those in the domiciliaries. Specifically, the nursing care unit residents tend to be drawn from better-educated individuals with more social resources; these residents are more impaired, have a lower activity level, and engage in fewer activities in the community. Although nursing care units have a higher staffing level than do domiciliaries, the two types of veterans facilities have similar scores on the Staff Resources subscale.

No direct comparison is possible between community and veterans facilities on the Social Resources subscale because one of the items, the percentage of residents receiving public assistance, is not applicable in veterans facilities. Compared with the community sample, residents of veterans facilities function somewhat more independently and are a bit more likely to participate in activities in the community. In addition, the domiciliary residents have a higher activity level than do those in

TABLE 3.4 RESIF Subscale Internal Consistency and Test-Retest Reliability

Subscale	Number of Items	Internal Consistency	Test-Retest Reliability (n = 12 Facilities)
Resident Social Resources	4	.68	.89
Resident Heterogeneity	10	.56	.68
Functional Abilities	15	.95	.99
Activity Level	13	.82	.95
Activities in the Community	14	.92	.99
Staff Resources	13	.71	.78

residential care facilities. The veterans facilities are also much higher than comparable community facilities on the Staff Resources subscale.

Subscale Internal Consistencies and Intercorrelations

Table 3.4 gives the number of items on each of the RESIF subscales and provides estimates of internal consistency (Cronbach's alpha). The alphas were calculated on a subset of the national sample because of missing data on some items and subscales. The number of facilities varied from more than 140 for Functional Abilities and Activity Level to 107 for Resident Social Resources and 106 for Resident Heterogeneity. In general, the internal consistencies are moderate to high. The limited number of items on the Resident Social Resources dimension is one factor contributing to its somewhat lower internal consistency.

The intercorrelations among the six subscales (partial correlations controlling for type of facility) for the community sample are shown above the diagonal in Table 3.5. The subscales were formulated so that each would tap a different area of functioning or set of characteristics. Although the subscales are thus conceptually distinct, they are empirically related. In particular, the three subscales measuring residents' current functioning are positively related. In facilities in which residents are more independent in daily living tasks, residents are also more likely to initiate activities in the facility and in the community. In general, however, the RESIF subscales show only moderate to low interrelationships. The intercorrelations for veterans facilities are shown below the diagonal in Table 3.5 and reflect a similar pattern.

TABLE 3.5 Partial Correlations Among RESIF Subscales, With Level of Care Controlled[a]

Subscale	Resident Social Resources	Resident Heterogeneity	Functional Abilities	Activity Level	Activities in the Community	Staff Resources
Resident Social Resources	—	.06	.07	.28	.15	.17
Resident Heterogeneity	.25	—	−.08	.04	.07	.10
Functional Abilities	−.26	.11	—	.42	.31	.01
Activity Level	−.25	−.01	.54	—	.46	.11
Activities in the Community	.06	.20	.44	.50	—	.06
Staff Resources	−.01	.11	.11	.02	.18	—

a. Correlations above the diagonal are for the community sample; correlations below the diagonal are for the veterans sample.

Test-Retest Reliability and Profile Stability

Subscale and profile stability data were obtained by readministering the RESIF in 12 facilities after an interval of 9 to 12 months. The test-retest results, shown in Table 3.4, indicate that the subscales have moderate to high test-retest reliability. Although functioning and activity levels may vary greatly for an individual over a year's time, these data indicate that the aggregate level of functioning for all individuals in a setting tends to remain remarkably constant, even with substantial resident turnover. We also computed the profile stability for each of the 12 facilities by calculating intraclass correlations on the RESIF standard scores for the two administrations in the facility. These correlations ranged from .73 to .98; 10 of the 12 correlations were above .80, confirming the pattern of relatively stable RESIF scores.

USING THE RESIF TO DESCRIBE GROUP RESIDENCES

The RESIF helps describe facilities, monitor program changes over time, and promote program improvement. When the RESIF is used with other parts of the Multiphasic Environmental Assessment Procedure (MEAP), it can help characterize the quality of a residential setting. Chapters 1 and 8 detail the applications of the MEAP. Here, we present RESIF profiles and illustrate how they can be used to describe facility residents and staff (for additional RESIF profiles, see Lemke & Moos, 1985; Moos & Lemke, 1994). The RESIF is most useful for such formative evaluations when results are compared with the appropriate normative sample.

Profile Interpretation

To illustrate the interpretation of facility profiles, we present RESIF profiles of three facilities in the community sample: a nursing home, a residential care facility, and a congregate apartment facility. These same three facilities are used to illustrate the other parts of the MEAP in Chapters 4 through 7. Results are shown as standard scores (based on the appropriate normative sample) with a mean of 50 and a standard deviation of 10.

City Haven Nursing Home

City Haven Nursing Home is located in an urban area on the west coast; when assessed, it had been owned and administered by a small corporation for less than a year following its purchase from an individual owner. As is typical of nursing homes in our sample, the majority of the 117 residents are over 80 years of age and are white (88%), widowed (64%) women (77%).

According to the RESIF profile shown in Figure 3.1, the residents are fairly typical for community nursing home residents in terms of their social resources, demographic diversity, and functional abilities. On the other hand, fewer residents take part in self-initiated activities or go into the community for activities than do residents in the average nursing home.

Not only is the staffing level lower than average (56 full-time staff for every 100 residents) but Staff Resources is low, due in part to the high staff turnover when the new owners took over.

El Dorado Residential Care Facility

El Dorado, housing 90 residents, is a moderate-sized residential care facility located in a suburban community on the west coast. The facility was constructed in the 1920s to serve an elderly population and has been run by the same nonprofit group since that time. El Dorado is a continuing care facility with a small nursing home attached. The facility

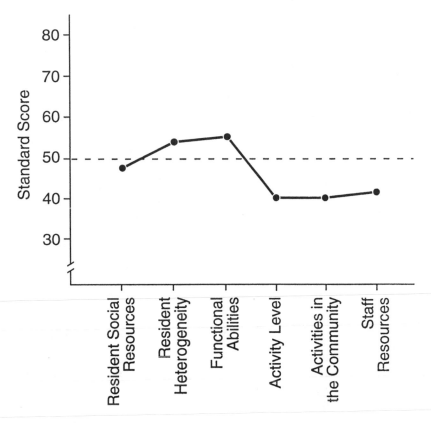

Figure 3.1. RESIF Profile for City Haven Nursing Home

charges a buy-in fee, but the fee is low enough to accommodate residents from a variety of backgrounds, and the endowment is adequate to cover residents with limited incomes.

Residents have quite low social resources (Figure 3.2); few residents completed any education beyond high school, and most held unskilled or blue-collar jobs or were full-time homemakers. More than half qualify for public assistance for low-income elderly people. The residents are a homogeneous group: Over 90% are women, three fourths are widowed, nearly all are white, and all are over age 75. With an average age of 86, residents are a substantially older group than those housed in most residential care facilities in which the average age is 79. Despite their

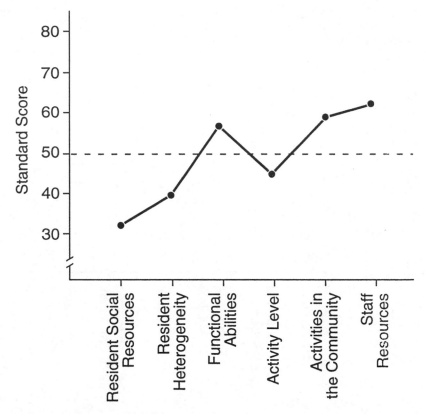

Figure 3.2. RESIF Profile for El Dorado Residential Care Facility

age, they are slightly more independent in daily activities and more active in the community than the average such resident group.

Although the staffing level is somewhat lower than average, with a ratio of 28 full-time equivalent (FTE) staff members for the 90 residents, staff are well trained, diverse in characteristics, and mostly long-term employees (high Staff Resources).

Marlborough Arms Apartments

Marlborough Arms, an apartment building housing about 50 residents, was constructed just 10 months before the assessment was carried out. Because of its recent construction, only about half the apartments

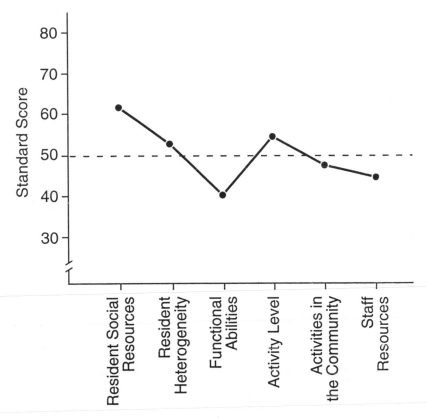

Figure 3.3. RESIF Profile for Marlborough Arms Apartments

were as yet occupied. Marlborough Arms is owned by a proprietary corporation that also runs nursing homes and residential care facilities; it is located in a suburban community in the northwest.

Marlborough Arms is not federally assisted housing, and its resident population consequently differs in certain respects from those typical of senior apartments (Figure 3.3). Residents have more social resources than average. Fewer residents are low-income elderly; only about 20% receive Supplemental Security Income. In addition, the resident group includes almost twice as many married couples as is typical. Averaging 81 years of age, residents are slightly older than apartment residents generally; they are also significantly more impaired. Their activity levels in the facility and in the community, however, are about average.

Although the staffing ratio is higher than that typically found in apartments because of low occupancy and high level of services, Staff Resources is about average. Not only are the staff all relatively new to their jobs, but they have no formal training program.

Monitoring Programs

The RESIF can be used to monitor a facility over time and to evaluate the results of independently initiated program modifications (e.g., Byerts & Heller, 1985). The RESIF is also useful in planning and evaluating interventions designed to change a facility (Wells & Singer, 1988; Wells, Singer, & Polgar, 1986).

For example, Hatcher, Gentry, Kunkel, and Smith (1983) used the RESIF and other parts of the MEAP to try to improve group homes for psychiatric clients. In one home, the RESIF showed that residents rarely participated in activities in the community. Project staff helped residents to organize meetings and to plan new activities. According to the RESIF, the intervention was successful: Residents' participation in community activities increased over time.

In another home, which housed men who had all had continuous psychiatric hospitalizations of 2 years or longer, the intervention focused on training the manager to increase his expectations and encourage residents to take more responsibility. House meetings were introduced to help the men confront household problems and plan group activities. On posttest, the RESIF showed substantial increases in residents' involvement in activities in the community. Residents also participated more in facility-planned activities.

More generally, the RESIF can help administrators understand the characteristics of the residents and staff in their facility, clarify how these characteristics affect facility goals, and suggest ways to improve specific aspects of the facility. Chapter 8 provides more information about these applications.

ADMINISTRATION OF THE RESIF

General Directions for the RESIF

The RESIF is contained in Appendix A; the scoring key is in Appendix B. To complete the RESIF, you will need to tabulate information from social histories, medical records, records of activities, and staff records. The number of residents determines how much time is needed to complete the RESIF; for 100 residents, allow about 3 hours to locate and tabulate information.

To organize your work, go through the form with the administrator, secretary, or head nurse and note the best source of information for each item. Then organize tally sheets on which you can group questions that will be answered from one source. For example, medical records may contain most of the information for Section I and some information for Section II; obtain all of this information at the same time so that you will not have to go through the same records twice.

In some cases, you may obtain information for a given section of the forms from a variety of sources. For example, you may have the Background Information Forms (BIF; see Appendix A) from half the residents, interviews with others, and a staff member's reports for the remainder. To keep track of your data collection in such cases, use a list of residents to check off the category of information as you obtain it.

Chapter 2 provides suggestions for presenting the MEAP to facility administrators and staff, setting policies about confidentiality and the use of results, and encouraging cooperation in the data collection process.

Multiunit Facilities

In multiunit facilities, you may need to prorate information for some sections (for details, see Defining the Unit in Chapter 2). Before starting data collection, clearly define the unit you want to study. Be sure that the administrator and other staff members respond to questions in terms of the unit under study.

Incomplete Data

Often, only part of the information for the RESIF can be obtained or information may be available on varying numbers of residents—for example, concerning their employment and education. Try to obtain the best estimate of the proportion of residents who fall into each category using the following guidelines:

1. Sometimes complete information is available on one category, but none is available on the others. For example, you may know exactly how many people are less than 55 years old but not how many of the

remainder fall into each category of those over age 55. In such cases, translate the known category into the percentage of total residents and leave the remaining categories blank (for missing information).

2. Similarly, you may be able to complete one category, but for the others you have information for only some of the residents. For example, in a facility with 50 residents, marital status may be known for everyone who is married (10 people) and for 20 additional people (of whom 3 are single, 5 are separated or divorced, and 12 are widowed). In such cases, translate the known category into the percentage of total residents and use the partial information for the other categories to make the best estimate you can. In the example just given, the married group represents 20% of the total resident group (10 of 50 people); therefore, count 20% as married. Categorize the remaining 80% of the residents into the other groups by using the available information on 20 people. There are 3 of 20 (15%) single people (15% × 80% = 12%); 5 of the 20 (25%) are separated or divorced (25% × 80% = 20%); and 12 of the 20 (60%) are widowed (60% × 80% = 48%). Note that the categories should total 100%: 20% + 12% + 20% + 48% = 100%.

3. In other cases, you may obtain information from records in which some information is missing for some residents. As a result, you may have a category of "unknown" that varies in size for different items. In such cases, you must decide whether the sample on whom you have information is fairly representative of the population of the facility as a whole; if it is, use the available data to estimate the characteristics of the whole. For example, if religion is missing from a number of records but no particular religious group is more likely than others to have this information missing, then the percentage of the sample in each category can be used to approximate the distribution for the residents as a whole. To calculate the percentage in each category, divide the number in each category (e.g., Catholic) by the number of residents for whom religion is known. For example, if religion is known for 25 residents in a 50-resident facility and 15 of the 25 are Catholic, then 15 ÷ 25 or 60% are Catholic. Again, note that the categories should total 100%.

4. If you can obtain information from records or from residents on only a small sample of residents, then estimates from staff members may be more accurate than estimates made on the basis of a sample. For example, classification into ethnic categories may not appear on any records, but knowledgeable staff members may be able to estimate this information fairly accurately.

All information on the number of residents or staff falling into particular categories should eventually be translated into percentages for purposes of scoring. Follow the guidelines previously mentioned. Check your calculations by adding the percentage of residents in each subcategory. For each item, the total should equal 100%. (Because of rounding, the total may actually range from about 98 to 102%.)

Scoring

Scoring can be completed using the reproducible worksheets in Appendix B. Appendix C contains directions for transforming raw percentage scores into standard scores for facility profiles. Allow an hour and a half to score and profile the RESIF.

Specific Directions for the RESIF

Section I: Residents' Background Characteristics

Information for this section may be obtained from various sources: admission and discharge records, medical records, or staff or resident reports. Some information (such as the number of residents, the number of men and women, or residents' ethnicity) may already be tabulated. If you are working from records, be sure to include only records of current residents. Some information may be more conveniently tabulated on specially designed sheets than directly on the form.

In facilities in which records on the residents are incomplete or nonexistent, have residents complete the Background Information Form (BIF; sample included in Appendix A); if you are also using the Sheltered Care Environment Scale (SCES), have residents complete the BIF and SCES at the same time. Try to obtain a high return rate; as needed, supplement this information with educated guesses from knowledgeable staff members. Some residents who are unable to complete the SCES may nevertheless be able to provide information about their backgrounds and activities if you use the BIF in an interview format.

Item 8: Occupation. Occupational level is based on the skill and authority associated with different occupations. The hierarchy ranges from unskilled physical labor to the more prestigious use of skill and the exercise of authority. Thus, a farmer might be classified in any category from unskilled to manager depending on the size, complexity, and value of the enterprise. The following examples help to define these categories (see also Duncan, 1961; Stevens & Featherman, 1981):

Unskilled—cafeteria worker, construction or general laborer, deckhand, domestic, farmhand, garbage collector, janitor, porter, shoeshine, stagehand, unemployed, unskilled factory worker, or window cleaner

Blue-collar (skilled manual workers, machine operators, and semiskilled workers)—assembly line worker, auto mechanic, baker, barber, bartender, butcher, carpenter, chef or cook, delivery person, driver, electrician, enlisted military personnel, firefighter, gardener, guard, hair stylist, heavy-equipment operator, hospital aide, lumberjack, machinist, mason, masseur or masseuse, mechanic, painter, plumber, postal worker, practical nurse, printer, repair person, small-scale farmer, tailor, waiter, or welder

Clerical/sales—bill collector, bookkeeper, claims examiner, clerk, employment interviewer, factory supervisor, farmer (large family farm), owner of one- to three-person business, or route manager

Semiprofessional—actor or theatrical producer, appraiser, commercial artist, court reporter, interior decorator, laboratory assistant, mortician, newspaper reporter, oral hygienist, photographer, surveyor, tool designer, or travel agent

Manager/managerial (administrative personnel or small business owner)—advertising, insurance, or purchasing agent; chief clerk; credit, service, shop, or store manager; farmer (corporate farm); government section head; insurance adjuster; owner of a four-person or larger business; private secretary; or sales representative

Executive/professional—accountant, agronomist, artist, auditor, bank officer, commissioned officer (lieutenant or above), dentist, economist, engineer, forester, government official, judge, lawyer, librarian, member of the clergy (professionally trained), musician, optician, personnel manager, pharmacist, physician, police chief, registered nurse, scientist, symphony conductor, or university professor

Homemaker—person not employed outside his or her own home

Item 10: Language. Include persons for whom English is a second language but only if their level of mastery prevents them from communicating effectively. Do not include those who are aphasic.

Item 11: Languages. This category can include more residents than those counted for Item 10—for example, those who are fluent in both English and another language.

Item 13b: Supplemental Security Income (SSI). This item refers to SSI (payments to low-income elderly persons) and not to regular social security payments.

Item 14: Other Forms of Aid. Other forms of aid include county or municipal aid and aid from nonprofit groups. Do not count social security or pensions.

Item 15: Length of Stay. Length of stay for residents who have entered the facility and have had a continuous stay can be tabulated by subtracting the date of admission or entrance from the present date. If a resident has entered the facility, left it for a time, and then reentered, determining length of stay poses a problem. The important factors in these cases are the length of absence and the reason for it. For example, a visit or vacation, whatever its length, would not be subtracted from the length of stay. In other cases, follow these guidelines:

1. absence for 1 week or less, whatever the reason—subtract the initial entrance date from the present date;
2. admission to hospital for illness—subtract the initial entrance date from the present date and subtract the length of hospitalization from this difference;
3. move to another residence (another nursing home, own apartment, or home)—calculate the length of stay from the most recent admission date.

Item 16: Preresidence Visit. What percentage of the residents (not their families) have an opportunity to look over the facility before moving in? This figure would not include those who move in at the same time they make their first visit. The prospective resident must have a real choice about whether to live in the facility.

Item 17: Deaths. Include all persons who have died in the facility or after a brief (3 days or less) hospital stay.

Item 18: Moving Away. Count the number of discharges in the preceding 3 months. If a resident goes to the hospital for a specific procedure (e.g., setting a broken bone or surgery) and is expected to return after the initial recovery period, do not count this as moving away. If rent is paid or a room is reserved for a person's return, again, do not count this as leaving. If a person leaves, however, intending at the time to make a permanent move, but later returns, count this as leaving.

Item 18a: Move to. Classify all persons counted in Item 18 into one of the categories. "Senior citizens apartments" includes federally funded congregate housing; a boarding home or residential care home offers some services, such as meals and housekeeping, but not 24-hour nursing care.

Section II: Residents' Functional Abilities

Depending on the level of functioning of residents, the extent of records, and the size of the facility, information on residents' functional abilities can be obtained from medical records, self-reports, knowledgeable staff members, or direct observation. In cases in which records do not contain information about functioning, rely on estimates from staff members or questions in the BIF. Note that Items 7 and 8 are not included in the BIF; this information must be obtained from another source. Tally sheets may be useful for organizing and carrying out the data collection.

Section II, Part I: Activities of Daily Living

Some items in Part I may be completed quickly in facilities that require a specific level of functioning for admission and continued residence. For example, if residents are required to be ambulatory without assistance, all residents could then be counted as having that ability. Simply because a facility does not provide assistance in a given task, however, does not mean that all residents can function independently. Remember that help may come from other residents, family members, or friends. To the extent possible, all such assistance should be included in evaluating functioning.

Task	Do this with some help	Unable to do this
2. Eat meals	Need help with eating	Tube- or spoon-fed
4. Walk	Use a walker or person's arm for support	Use a wheelchair or bedridden
5. Get in and out of bed	Need help getting in or out of bed	Bedridden
7. Get to bathroom	May need reminder or occasionally incontinent	Consistently incontinent, catheterized
8. Needs understood	Person somewhat confused or ability to communicate impaired	Person usually confused or ability to communicate seriously impaired

Task	Do this with some help	Unable to do this
9. Handle money	Facility, friends, or family helps with bills, banking	Someone else handles all bills, banking, and so on
10. Telephone	May need help finding or dialing number	Can neither find number nor dial it

Section III: Participation in Activities Outside the Facility

This information may be obtained from a knowledgeable staff member or from the BIF. In the former case, you may obtain overall estimates in a large facility or you may check off activity participation on a list of residents in a small facility. Count only those activities that take residents off the facility grounds. For example, if residents attend services in the facility's chapel, attendance should not be counted here.

Section IV, Characteristics of Staff and Volunteers, Part I: Staff

To collect some of the information in Part I, you will need to tabulate information from personnel records. To determine the number of FTE staff, use an information sheet with the number of hours each individual works in a week; payroll records can also be helpful. To calculate the FTE for part-time staff, divide by 40 the number of hours an individual works in a week. If hourly totals are listed by classification (e.g., total RN hours), divide this total by 40 to calculate the number of staff FTE. For Part I, Items 3 and 4, tabulate information from staff employment records. Record the information on tally sheets or directly on the form.

Items 1 and 2: Staff FTEs. List only those staff members who are hired or contracted by the facility. Do not include public health nurses who visit once a week as part of their district responsibility or physicians who visit private patients. Physician owners count as medical staff only if they provide medical care to the residents.

In multiunit facilities in which one or a few units are being assessed, count only those staff members who are functionally available to the residents in the units being assessed; count these staff only in terms of the FTE hours they are available to those residents. Consider, for example, a facility in which the residential care unit is being assessed but the nursing home is not. If some registered nurses (RNs) from the nursing home make daily visits to supervise medications in the residential care unit, record the FTE hours the RNs are functionally available to those in the residential care unit.

Items 3 and 4: Length of Employment and Staff Characteristics. These questions apply to all staff members currently employed.

Item 5a: Other Languages. For the staff members who give direct service to residents and fluently speak languages other than English, list the languages and the number of staff members who speak each language.

Item 6a: In-Service Training. Check the category that best characterizes the in-service training provided to the staff. Give credit for the highest level of training provided.

4

PHYSICAL AND ARCHITECTURAL FEATURES CHECKLIST

The Physical and Architectural Features Checklist (PAF) measures the physical resources of group residential settings for older people. It comprises 153 scored items that cover facility location, physical features inside and outside the facility, and space allowances. The PAF focuses on the availability of these resources and not on their use. A set of 31 additional items provide descriptive information about the neighborhood and building. All information is obtained by direct observation.

The PAF measures the actual resources in a facility. We have also adapted the PAF to assess individuals' preferences for physical resources in a facility (PAF Form I).

PAF SUBSCALES

The eight PAF subscales are presented in Table 4.1. The first subscale, Community Accessibility, measures the facility's proximity to resources in the community; it reflects the degree of physical integration between the facility and surrounding community and indicates how easily residents can use local services.

49

TABLE 4.1 Physical and Architectural Features (PAF) Subscale Descriptions

Subscale	Description
	Degree of physical integration
Community Accessibility	Extent to which the community and its services are convenient and accessible
	Physical features for comfort and involvement
Physical Amenities	Physical features that add convenience, attractiveness, and comfort
Social-Recreational Aids	Physical features that foster social interaction and recreational activities
	Supportive physical features
Prosthetic Aids	Extent to which the facility provides a barrier-free environment and aids to physical independence and mobility
Orientational Aids	Extent to which the setting provides features that help orient residents
Safety Features	Extent to which communal areas can be monitored; the presence of features for preventing accidents
	Space for resident and staff functions
Staff Facilities	Physical facilities that aid the staff and make it pleasant for them to maintain and manage the setting
Space Availability	Number and size of communal areas in relation to the number of residents; size allowances for personal space

The next two subscales, Physical Amenities and Social-Recreational Aids, focus on the presence of physical features that improve comfort and foster activities.

The next three subscales assess supportive physical features. Prosthetic Aids measures the provision of aids to physical independence and mobility; Orientational Aids measures the presence of features that help orient the resident to time, place, and persons; and Safety Features assesses the availability of features to prevent intrusions and accidents.

The last two subscales assess the allowance of space for resident and staff functions. Staff Facilities taps the presence of physical features that make the setting more pleasant for staff. This dimension is included because such features may enhance staff performance and contribute to the quality of resident care. Space Availability reflects the communal and personal space available to residents.

NORMATIVE SAMPLES AND
PSYCHOMETRIC CHARACTERISTICS

Normative Samples

Normative data for the PAF are available from two samples of facilities for older adults: 262 community facilities and 81 facilities serving veterans (see Normative Samples in Chapter 1).

Most PAF items allow for a dichotomous response, reflecting the presence or absence of a particular feature. Scoring of some items on the Space Availability subscale requires transformation of nondichotomous responses, such as square-footage allowances, into dichotomous distributions. The cutoff points for these items were established on the basis of conceptual criteria and the actual distributions obtained from our sample of facilities.

The raw scores for a facility are percentage scores reflecting the number of features present out of the total number possible. For example, the Physical Amenities subscale of the PAF asks about the presence in the facility of 30 features that contribute to making the facility more comfortable. Facility scores can vary from 0% to 100%. A facility that has 15 of the 30 physical features obtains a raw score of 50%. The average score for the total community sample on Physical Amenities is 64%. Each of the means and standard deviations in Table 4.2 was derived in a similar way.

The PAF itself is in Appendix A, hand-scoring worksheets are in Appendix B, and tables for converting raw percentage scores to standard scores are in Appendix C.

Community Facilities

Means and standard deviations for the eight PAF subscales for the total community sample and for each of the three subsamples are reported in Table 4.2. The sample of community facilities varied considerably on all eight subscales, as shown by the standard deviations in Table 4.2. For example, scores on Community Accessibility ranged from 0% to 100%. The variation of scores within each of the three types of facilities is similar in magnitude to the overall sample variation for all but the Prosthetic Aids subscale. This pattern indicates that the PAF dimensions are sensitive to the differences among facilities of a given type.

The norms for the three types of community facilities reflect meaningful variations between types of residential settings related to such

TABLE 4.2 PAF Subscale Means and Standard Deviations for the Total Community Sample and the Three Subsamples

Subscale	Total Sample (n = 262 Facilities)		Nursing Homes (n = 135 Facilities)		Residential Care (n = 60 Facilities)		Apartments (n = 67 Facilities)	
	Mean	SD	Mean	SD	Mean	SD	Mean	SD
Community Accessibility	49	25	43	25	49	25	60	20
Physical Amenities	64	14	65	12	62	16	63	14
Social-Recreational Aids	63	15	64	14	63	17	62	16
Prosthetic Aids	65	17	77	9	52	18	53	11
Orientational Aids	50	14	53	13	43	16	51	14
Safety Features	68	16	69	15	63	18	71	17
Staff Facilities	57	24	67	18	48	31	46	21
Space Availability	51	22	45	22	63	20	51	21

factors as the impairment of their residents, their staffing levels, and the degree of regulation under which they function. For example, of the three types, nursing homes have the highest average scores on Prosthetic Aids and Staff Facilities, features appropriate to their impaired residents and high staffing levels. Factors such as the age of their buildings, their smaller size, and the absence of uniform regulation, appear to contribute to the finding that residential care facilities have fewer orientational aids and safety features but more space for residents than do the other types of facilities. Congregate apartments are more likely to be in multistory buildings; as a consequence, they tend to be located in more densely developed neighborhoods and to have better community accessibility.

Veterans Facilities

The PAF means and standard deviations for the sample of 81 veterans facilities and for each of the two subsamples are given in Table 4.3. As in the community sample, there is considerable variability among facilities on all eight subscales. For example, facility scores on Community Accessibility range from 6% to 94%. The variability of scores within each of the two types of veterans facilities is also fairly substantial, indicating that the PAF dimensions are sensitive to the differences among each type of veterans facilities.

TABLE 4.3 PAF Subscale Means and Standard Deviations for the Total
Veterans Sample and the Two Subsamples

Subscale	Total Sample (n = 81 Facilities)		Nursing Care Units (n = 57 Facilities)		Domiciliaries (n = 24 Facilities)	
	Mean	*SD*	*Mean*	*SD*	*Mean*	*SD*
Community Accessibility	37	24	39	23	34	26
Physical Amenities	70	15	70	16	71	13
Social-Recreational Aids	72	14	69	14	77	13
Prosthetic Aids	71	14	73	12	66	16
Orientational Aids	49	14	48	12	52	17
Safety Features	58	15	60	14	54	18
Staff Facilities	63	21	63	21	63	23
Space Availability	65	17	66	18	62	17

The two types of veterans facilities provide similar physical environments, but compared with the domiciliaries the veterans nursing care
units tend to provide somewhat more prosthetic aids and somewhat
fewer social-recreational aids.

Compared with the community nursing homes, the veterans nursing
care units have more physical amenities, social-recreational aids, and
space availability but fewer prosthetic aids and safety features. The
domiciliaries provide more social-recreational aids, prosthetic aids, and
staff facilities than do residential care facilities. On the other hand,
domiciliaries have somewhat fewer safety features and less community
accessibility than do residential care facilities.

Subscale Internal Consistencies
and Intercorrelations

Table 4.4 shows the number of items on each of the PAF subscales and
provides estimates of internal consistency (Cronbach's alpha). Most of
the alphas are based on data from more than 140 facilities in the
community sample, but because some data were missing and some items
did not apply to all facilities a reduced set of facilities was used for
calculating the internal consistency of some dimensions. Because types
of facilities vary in how they organize public and private space, the alpha
for Space Availability was calculated separately for the nursing home and

TABLE 4.4 PAF Subscale Internal Consistency and Test-Retest Reliability

Subscale	Number of Items	Internal Consistency	Test-Retest Reliability ($n = 12$ Facilities)
Community Accessibility	16	.84	.89[a]
Physical Amenities	30	.71	.88
Social-Recreational Aids	28	.73	.75
Prosthetic Aids	24	.82	.95
Orientational Aids	13	.62	.61
Safety Features	18	.71	.76
Staff Facilities	11	.81	.79
Space Availability	13	.66	.95

a. $n = 9$ facilities.

residential care facilities (alpha = .59) and apartments (alpha = .72); then the alphas were averaged to provide one estimate of internal consistency.

In general, the internal consistencies are reasonably high, especially considering that most PAF subscales cover a wide array of physical features. For example, the Orientational Aids subscale comprises a particularly diverse set of items dealing with orientation to time, place, and person. Although all of the items tap aspects of orientation, the internal consistency of the subscale is moderate because item relationships are relatively low.

The intercorrelations among the eight subscales (partial correlations controlling for level of care) for the community sample are shown above the diagonal in Table 4.5. Overall, the subscale intercorrelations are relatively low (average $r = .28$). The correlations among the last seven PAF subscales are positive; thus, a facility with more resources in one area tends to have more resources in other areas, particularly for physical amenities, social-recreational aids, and staff facilities. These relationships are moderate, however, indicating that the subscales measure somewhat independent aspects of a facility's physical resources.

Subscale intercorrelations for the veterans facilities, shown below the diagonal in Table 4.5, tend to be somewhat lower than those for the community normative sample; they provide additional support for the conclusion that the subscales tap somewhat distinct aspects of a facility's physical environment.

TABLE 4.5 Partial Correlations Among PAF Subscales, With Level of Care Controlled[a]

Subscale	Community Accessibility	Physical Amenities	Social-Recreational Aids	Prosthetic Aids	Orientational Aids	Safety Features	Staff Facilities	Space Availability
Community Accessibility	—	−.06	.07	.03	.03	.18	.08	−.11
Physical Amenities	.17	—	.57	.40	.37	.32	.54	.37
Social-Recreational Aids	−.19	.43	—	.25	.32	.34	.52	.38
Prosthetic Aids	.22	.49	.38	—	.40	.31	.45	.02
Orientational Aids	−.04	.23	.08	.27	—	.42	.38	.05
Safety Features	−.16	.07	.39	.13	.24	—	.39	.14
Staff Facilities	.06	.15	.36	.09	.10	.32	—	.24
Space Availability	−.13	−.06	.20	−.04	.13	.21	.17	—

a. Correlations above the diagonal are for the community sample; correlations below the diagonal are for the veterans sample.

Interobserver Reliability, Test-Retest Reliability, and Profile Stability

To obtain interobserver reliability data for the PAF, two project observers, two staff members, and two community residents independently completed the PAF in 15 facilities (7 nursing homes, 4 residential care facilities, and 4 congregate apartments). The results indicate that trained observers can provide reliable ratings on most of the PAF subscales; interobserver reliability was above .70 on six of the subscales. It was only moderate, however, on Physical Amenities ($r = .55$) and Safety Features ($r = .61$).

Scores from staff members show lower agreement with project observer scores, but the average of their ratings is a reliable estimate except for Orientational Aids and Staff Facilities. Two community observers averaging their independent results or arriving at a consensus produce a very reliable rating of the facility's physical resources (for guidelines on recommended training for observers, see Administration of the PAF).

Subscale and profile stability data were obtained by completing the PAF in 12 of these facilities after an interval of 9 to 12 months. The test-retest results, shown in Table 4.4, indicate that with the exception of Orientational Aids, the PAF scores are relatively stable over time. The low test-retest correlation for Orientational Aids occurs despite a very high interrater reliability, suggesting that facilities underwent actual change and that these features may be more easily altered than the others.

The profile stability for each of the 12 facilities in the test-retest sample was computed by calculating intraclass correlations on the PAF standard scores for the two administrations in the facility. These correlations ranged from .51 to .96. The low-profile stability correlation occurred in a facility that occupied a relatively new building and experienced an increase in Social-Recreational Aids from 46% to 75% as new furnishings were acquired. Correlations for 8 of the 12 facilities were above .80, confirming the pattern of relatively stable PAF scores.

THE IDEAL FORM

The Ideal Form of the PAF (PAF Form I) measures individuals' preferences for physical features of group residential facilities. Form I parallels the PAF, except that it has seven dimensions; we did not include the Space Availability subscale in Form I because we were not able to develop a simple method to assess preferences for space allowances. Form I has 140 items, each of which is parallel to an item on the PAF.

Development

We developed the PAF Form I by rewording PAF items to elicit information about individual preferences. Thus, for example, the PAF item "Are there handrails in the halls?" (a prosthetic feature) was reworded as "Should there be handrails in the halls?" We tried to keep the individual items as simple as possible and, to facilitate administration of Form I in a written questionnaire or interview format, worded all items as questions. The items are answered on a 4-point scale varying from "not important" to "desirable," "very important," and "essential." After a series of item trials and revisions, we constructed a version of the PAF Form I composed of seven of the eight PAF subscales (for more details, see Brennan, Moos, & Lemke, 1988).

The PAF Form I was administered to nine groups of respondents ($n = 799$) along with a questionnaire covering sociodemographic and personal characteristics. The respondents included (a) older people living in nursing homes, residential care facilities, and congregate apartments; (b) staff working in nursing homes, residential care facilities, and congregate apartments; (c) older people who were living in an apartment facility and were asked to answer in terms of a new nursing home; (d) older people living independently who were asked to envision an ideal group residence for semi-independent elderly; and (e) gerontologists who were experts on residential settings for older people.

Because the PAF Form I helps people describe the type of facility they would like, it can facilitate comparisons of the preferences of administrators, staff, residents, potential residents, and experts. It can also reveal individual variations in preferences, which should be considered when planning residential settings for heterogeneous groups of older people.

Used with the PAF, Form I helps to measure person-environment congruence by contrasting the preferences of current or potential residents with the actual qualities of a setting. It can thus identify areas in which respondents want change. (For further details on potential applications, see Brennan et al., 1988; Moos & Lemke, 1984, 1994; Moos, Lemke, & Clayton, 1983; Moos, Lemke, & David, 1987.)

The PAF Form I and scoring directions are provided in Appendix D.

Normative Samples

The means and standard deviations of the PAF Form I subscales are shown in Table 4.6 for residents, Table 4.7 for staff, and Table 4.8 for potential residents and experts. The scores are given in terms of the percentage of items rated very important or essential by the average respondent. This dichotomous scoring system facilitates comparisons between individual preferences and characteristics of actual facilities because all PAF items are scored dichotomously. A 4-point scoring system (varying from 0 for not important to 3 for essential) results in roughly comparable percentage means and standard deviations; investigators who wish to use the 4-point scoring system can compare their results with the means and standard deviations given in Appendix D.

Using dichotomous scoring, an individual who rates 8 of the 16 Community Accessibility items as very important or essential obtains a score of 50%. The average endorsement rate on Community Accessibility was 50% for the 422 residents, 45% for staff, and 54% for experts, as

TABLE 4.6 PAF Form I Subscale Means and Standard Deviations for the
Total Sample and the Three Subsamples of Residents

Subscale	Total Sample of Residents (n = 422)		Nursing Home Residents (n = 40)		Residential Care Residents (n = 153)		Apartment Residents (n = 229)	
	Mean	SD	Mean	SD	Mean	SD	Mean	SD
Community Accessibility	50	27	33	28	54	28	49	25
Physical Amenities	47	21	48	19	51	25	44	19
Social-Recreational Aids	37	21	42	19	40	26	34	18
Prosthetic Aids	55	22	73	16	60	24	50	20
Orientational Aids	49	23	47	20	51	26	48	21
Safety Features	66	23	66	17	66	26	66	21
Staff Facilities	41	31	54	26	48	36	35	27

shown in Tables 4.6, 4.7, and 4.8. Each of the means and standard deviations in Tables 4.6, 4.7, and 4.8 was derived in the same way. The standard deviations indicate that all groups had substantial individual differences in preferences.

Relative Importance of Physical Features

Based on the average ratings, the seven PAF Form I subscales can be ranked in order of their relative importance to residents. Safety Features received the highest overall rating, followed by Prosthetic Aids, Community Accessibility, and Orientational Aids. Physical Amenities, Staff Facilities, and Social-Recreational Aids received slightly lower overall ratings.

Residents had nearly unanimous preferences for such safety features as adequate lighting in outside areas and on steps, nonslip surfaces in appropriate places, smoke detectors, and call buttons in living areas and bathrooms. Older people have strong preferences for physical features that aid them in negotiating the facility environment. Most residents of group living settings prefer such prosthetic aids as reserved parking for handicapped people, handrails in the hallways and bathrooms, lift bars next to the toilet, and wheelchair access. A smaller but still substantial proportion of residents want the front door to open and close automat-

TABLE 4.7 PAF Form I Subscale Means and Standard Deviations for the
Total Sample and the Three Subsamples of Staff

Subscale	Total Sample of Staff (n = 98)		Nursing Home Staff (n = 33)		Residential Care Staff (n = 34)		Apartment Staff (n = 31)	
	Mean	SD	Mean	SD	Mean	SD	Mean	SD
Community Accessibility	45	23	43	29	42	24	49	14
Physical Amenities	57	21	63	22	58	18	51	20
Social-Recreational Aids	49	23	54	26	48	22	46	22
Prosthetic Aids	61	19	70	16	58	20	56	20
Orientational Aids	53	22	57	25	50	22	50	20
Safety Features	71	18	72	17	71	18	68	18
Staff Facilities	65	30	76	28	63	32	57	27

ically, to have handrails in apartment areas, and to have such bathroom features as a flexible shower and shower seats. Residents also strongly prefer such orientational aids as a reception desk and a conveniently located bulletin board.

Although social-recreational aids emerged as the least important of the seven types of features, more than 50% of the respondents in residential settings strongly desire adequate parking for visitors, seating in the lobby, a comfortably furnished lounge or community room near the entrance, a patio or open courtyard, and a piano or organ (for more details, see Brennan et al., 1988; Moos et al., 1987).

Differences Among Resident and Staff Groups

The data show substantial differences among subgroups of residents and staff. For example, residents in nursing homes prefer more prosthetic aids compared with residents in the other types of facilities, but they feel that community accessibility is less important. Nursing home residents are also more likely to endorse the importance of facilities for staff.

When older people living in congregate apartments (potential residents) describe the ideal nursing home, the descriptions are similar to the views of current nursing home residents, except that potential

TABLE 4.8   PAF Form I Subscale Means and Standard Deviations for
Potential Residents and Experts

Subscale	Potential Nursing Home Residents (n = 30)		Potential Apartment Residents (n = 205)		Experts Describing Apartments (n = 44)	
	Mean	SD	Mean	SD	Mean	SD
Community Accessibility	51	25	49	23	54	18
Physical Amenities	44	20	48	22	67	16
Social-Recreational Aids	37	23	36	22	52	20
Prosthetic Aids	69	25	61	22	76	15
Orientational Aids	45	23	47	25	61	24
Safety Features	69	19	69	22	76	16
Staff Facilities	48	36	36	33	53	28

residents view community accessibility as more important than do current residents. Older people living in the community (potential residents)
generally agree with current residents in their preferences concerning
congregate apartments, although the potential residents have somewhat stronger preferences for prosthetic aids.

Compared with staff in residential care facilities and apartments, staff
in nursing homes prefer more physical amenities and staff facilities.
Compared with residents in comparable types of facilities, staff members
generally feel that more physical features are very important or essential.
Similarly, gerontological experts, who rated apartment facilities, rate
every dimension except staff facilities higher than do current apartment
residents and staff. In particular, they have stronger preferences for
physical amenities, prosthetic aids, and orientational aids.

Subscale internal Consistencies
and Intercorrelations

The PAF Form I subscale internal consistencies (Cronbach's alpha)
were calculated on the overall sample of 799 respondents; all are
relatively high ($r = .78$ and above). The intercorrelations among the
seven PAF Form I subscales are all moderate to high for residents, staff,
and experts. The relatively high subscale intercorrelations suggest that
there are consistent individual preference patterns that apply across all

dimensions. For example, individual residents and staff who express a preference for many physical amenities also tend to prefer more social-recreational aids and orientational aids. In contrast, the associations among PAF subscales are only moderate, as shown in Table 4.5. These findings point to the fact that although the PAF Form I does not require respondents to establish priorities among physical features, most congregate facilities must do so in actual practice.

USING THE PAF TO
DESCRIBE GROUP RESIDENCES

The PAF has been used widely in characterizing facilities and evaluating programs. It helps to describe facilities, to monitor program changes over time, and to promote program improvement. When the PAF and the PAF Form I are both used, they can alert administrators to discrepancies between a facility's features and resident or staff preferences. When the PAF is used with other Multiphasic Environmental Assessment Procedure (MEAP) instruments, it can help characterize the quality of a residential setting. Chapters 1 and 8 describe in detail the applications of the MEAP.

Profile Interpretation

The PAF can be used to provide a systematic description of the physical resources available within a facility. The PAF is most useful for such formative evaluations when results are expressed in terms of the conditions that generally prevail in the appropriate normative sample.

To illustrate the interpretation of facility profiles, we present PAF profiles of the three community facilities introduced in Chapter 3. Results are shown as standard scores with a mean of 50 and a standard deviation of 10. (For additional examples of PAF profiles, see Lemke & Moos, 1985; Moos & Lemke, 1994; Moos et al., 1987; Timko & Moos, 1991a.)

City Haven Nursing Home

Figure 4.1 shows the PAF profile for City Haven Nursing Home. Because of its urban location, City Haven is close to more community resources than the average nursing home (high Community Accessibil-

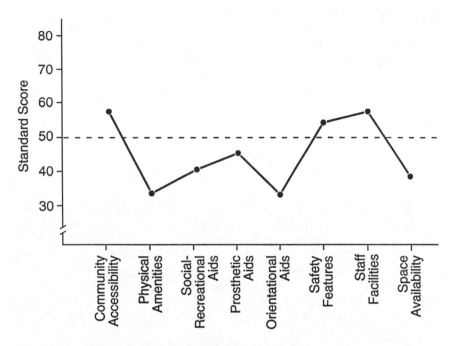

Figure 4.1. PAF Profile for City Haven Nursing Home

ity). It also scores high on Staff Facilities because most of the lower floor is devoted to office space, a staff meeting room, and a staff lounge. This facility receives low scores on Physical Amenities (e.g., it lacks landscaping and sheltered outside areas and the rooms do not have mirrors or individual temperature controls), Social-Recreational Aids (e.g., no outside seating, sparsely furnished patios, and no TV or radio in the communal areas), and Orientational Aids (e.g., no reception desk, corridors not color coded, and complex floor plan). The low score on Space Availability suggests that the ample provision of staff facilities may have been attained at some cost to the space available to residents.

El Dorado Residential Care Facility

The PAF profile for El Dorado is shown in Figure 4.2. When compared with other residential care facilities, El Dorado provides a very rich physical environment for its residents. It is close to a large number of community facilities including a grocery store, drugstore, church, bank, and park. It provides a large number of features to ensure comfort (including such features as a sheltered entrance, air-conditioning, a chapel, community kitchen, laundry room, and both a shower and bathtub for each resident) and to support activity and social interaction (such as a garden area for residents, a library, a music room, and lounges furnished with writing desks and small tables). Space for residents and staff is ample, and many features help ensure the safety and security of residents. The building entrance is well lighted, outside seating and the entry can be monitored from offices and public areas, only one entrance is left unlocked and it is monitored by a staff member, halls are equipped with smoke detectors, and residents' rooms have call buttons.

The building has only the average number of features to aid those with physical disabilities in part because of the less stringent building requirements in effect in the 1920s. For example, the halls are only six feet wide and have no handrails, bathrooms and showers cannot accommodate wheelchairs, drinking fountains are not accessible to wheelchairs, and the public phones have no volume control for hearing-impaired persons. The building also is about average in features designed to orient residents to their surroundings. Residents' names are on their doors and there is a public bulletin board, but the building is not color coded and the public area does not have posted lists of staff or residents or a map of community resources.

El Dorado thus provides a comfortable and stimulating environment. Residents take advantage of its location by involving themselves in a variety of community activities. Within the facility, the residents' activity level is just average despite the features designed to support such activities. Consistent with the fact that facility residents are relatively independent in daily activities, El Dorado has only an average number of supportive features.

Marlborough Arms Apartments

Figure 4.3, the PAF profile for Marlborough Arms, indicates that the physical environment is fairly typical of senior apartments. The facility does offer much more space than most; even at full occupancy, it would provide more communal and personal space than most apartment buildings. In contrast, very little space is devoted to staff functions, even though the staffing level is higher than average.

Marlborough Arms offers somewhat more than average physical amenities such as a sheltered entrance, furnished patio, air-conditioning, gift shop and laundry room, and drinking fountains and phones in public

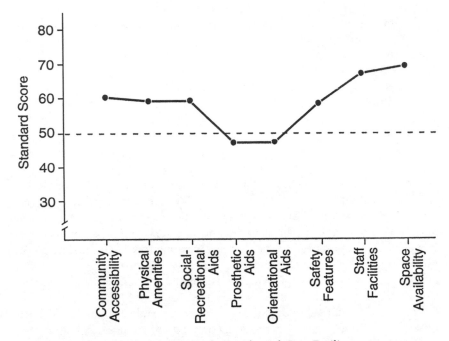

Figure 4.2. PAF Profile for El Dorado Residential Care Facility

areas. On the other hand, it has somewhat fewer features to support social and recreational activities. For example, it does not have a garden area for resident use, a library, a piano or organ, or a stereo system—features that are offered by the majority of apartments. Other features are all close to the average for apartments.

Thus, Marlborough Arms reflects the conditions available in most apartment facilities, except that it has much greater space allowances for residents and much less for staff. There is slightly more emphasis on comfort and slightly less on stimulating activity than in the average congregate apartment facility.

Monitoring Facilities and Guiding Interventions

Closely related to its use as a descriptive tool, the PAF can be used to measure a facility over time and to document the changes that occur in

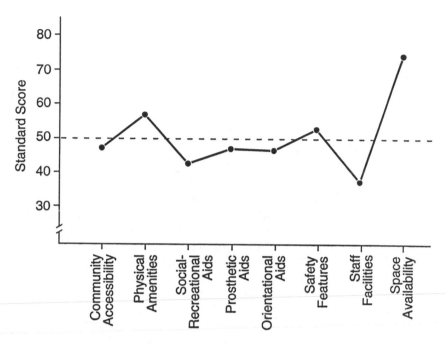

Figure 4.3. PAF Profile for Marlborough Arms Apartments

the physical environment. In addition, the PAF can help to identify problem areas, guide improvements, and monitor the impact of interventions. The PAF enables administrators and staff to understand the physical environment in their facility, to clarify how these resources serve resident and staff needs, and to suggest ways to improve specific aspects of the facility (see Chapters 1 and 8).

Comparing Actual and Preferred Physical Features

Information about preferences can help in identifying problems, planning interventions, matching residents with facilities, and understanding the perspectives of different interest groups. Kodama (1988a, 1988b) used a Japanese version of the PAF and found that residents' complaints about physical features were predictably related to the actual physical features in their facilities. That is, the fewer physical amenities, social-recreational aids, and so on, the higher the number of complaints in these specific areas.

Preferences of Apartment Residents

To illustrate these ideas, we compare the actual features of Marlborough Arms with a description of the ideal congregate apartment. The ideal profile presented in Figure 4.4 is based on PAF Form I responses of the normative group of congregate apartment residents (also shown in Table 4.6). Similar comparisons can be made with the preferences of an individual respondent such as a current or prospective resident. In the figure, each real and ideal subscale score is presented as a percentage score. The open bar represents the actual environment of Marlborough Arms, and the darkened area represents preferences in terms of the percentage of items rated as very important or essential.

Marlborough Arms generally has the number of physical features desired by the average apartment resident. For example, Marlborough Arms has 73% of the possible physical amenities and, on average, apartment residents rated 44% of them as very important or essential (also see Table 4.6). In only one area—staff facilities—does Marlborough Arms not meet the ideal. The facility also compares well with the ideal as defined by older people currently living in their own homes (Table 4.8); Marlborough Arms meets or exceeds their ideal in all areas except prosthetic aids and staff facilities.

Another way to compare real and ideal physical features is to determine whether a facility provides key features, defined as those rated very important or essential by a given percentage of respondents. For example, one might determine that if at least 25% of respondents rate an item very important, it should be considered a key feature.

Such a comparison shows that Marlborough Arms has most of the specific physical amenities, social-recreational aids, and safety features desired by at least 25% of apartment residents in the normative group. Among the key features it lacks are individual heating and air-conditioning controls, weather protection for the main entrance, choice of large or small tables for meals, and access to a library area and piano. Respondents would also like to see monitoring of the entry areas and nonslip surfaces on stairs and bathroom floors. Similarly, Marlborough Arms lacks some specific prosthetic aids, orientational aids, and staff facilities that at least a minority of apartment residents view as very important.

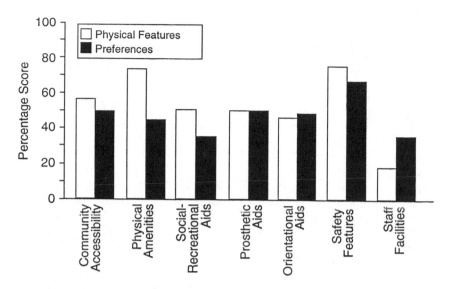

Figure 4.4. Physical Features in Marlborough Arms and Preferences of Apartment Residents

ADMINISTRATION OF THE PAF

General Directions for the PAF

A trained observer can complete the PAF using direct observation and measurement supplemented by information from the administrator or a staff member familiar with the facility. For training, an observer should complete practice assessments in at least three facilities and review the results, including discussion and resolution of discrepancies, with a second observer. Facility staff and community residents can complete the PAF using the directions that follow; reliability improves if the results from two observers are averaged or if the observers resolve discrepancies by mutual agreement.

The PAF is divided into sections arranged in logical order for data collection, although this order may need to be adapted to the particular facility. Allow 2 to 4 hours to complete the PAF in the average-sized facility. Arrange to collect data at a time appropriate to the facility and convenient for the administrator or staff member who will answer your questions and give you access to several resident rooms or apartments.

Try to complete the entire PAF without assistance, then review unanswered questions with an administrator or staff member.

Chapter 2 provides suggestions for presenting the MEAP to facility
administrators and staff, setting policies about confidentiality and the use
of results, and encouraging cooperation in the data collection process.

Making Measurements

To make measurements, you will need a blueprint, a floor plan with
room measurements on it, a fixed extendable tape measure, or a plain
tape measure and an assistant to hold one end. For tiled floors, which
come in standard 9- or 12-inch squares, you can count the tiles and
multiply by their dimension.

Multiunit Facilities

In multiunit facilities, the unit being studied may share physical
resources with other units. Credit the unit with any physical or architectural feature to which residents have access, and calculate space availability in terms of the per person square footage available to potential
users. For example, a 20-acre facility may have 500 residents, of which
50 are in the unit being studied. For the acreage allowance on the PAF,
first compute the overall acreage per person (20 acres per 500 residents
or .04 acre per resident) and then multiply by the number of people in
the target unit (50 residents × .04 acre per resident = 2 acres for the
target unit).

Use similar reasoning to count the number of lounges, special activity
areas, or dining areas. For example, suppose that three lounges in a
central building are available to 500 residents, and two lounges are in
the building being studied and are thus shared by only 50 residents. To
arrive at the number of lounges available to the residents of the building,
credit them with their share of the joint lounges (3 lounges ÷ 500
residents × 50 residents = .3) and with the two lounges that belong
exclusively to the unit for a total of 2.3 lounges.

Not Applicable Items

All items apply to all facilities except where specifically noted under
the directions for individual questions. The following examples illustrate

the rationale used to determine whether an item can be considered "not applicable."

For most items, their presence is an asset and their absence is a liability that detracts from a characteristic of the physical environment. For example, the Physical Amenities subscale includes the question "Is it [the seating in front of the building] protected from the weather?" This question is applicable in all cases whether or not there is seating. If there is no outside seating at all (or if this seating is not protected from the weather), this item should be marked "no." Protected seating near the entrance is a physical amenity that can be provided in any type of facility. The absence of outside seating that is protected diminishes the number of physical amenities a facility provides.

In contrast, items that can be considered not applicable contribute to an aspect of the physical environment, but their absence does not detract from it. For example, the item "Is it [the outside seating in front of the building] visible from the office or station of an employee?" is not applicable in those facilities in which there is no such seating. This is because the issue of safety (visibility to staff) does not arise if there is no outside seating. Similarly, if there are stairs, then nonskid surfaces contribute to their safety; if there are no stairs (and hence no nonskid surfaces), however, the facility safety is not affected.

Scoring

Hand scoring can be accomplished using the reproducible worksheets in Appendix B. Allow an hour and a half to score and profile the PAF.

Directions for the PAF Form I

Suggestions for administering the PAF-I to residents and staff are provided in Chapter 2. The PAF Form I and its scoring instructions are available in Appendix D.

Specific Directions for the PAF

Section I: Neighborhood Context

You can observe most of the Section I items from a brief tour of the grounds and neighborhood. To help you complete this section, use a map of the area. On the map, draw a circle with a 1/4-mile radius and the facility at the center; become familiar with this area.

Item 1: Urban, Suburban, or Rural Neighborhood. Assess the population density of the neighborhood within 1/4 mile of the facility. If it is sparsely populated with a fair amount of farming or open land, it is a rural area. If houses and commercial structures are quite close together but maintain separate yards and there are few or no large tracts of open land or farms, it is a suburban area. If houses have small or no yards and the majority of structures are multifamily housing, high-rise apartments, and commercial structures, the area is urban. Consider the entire area within the 1/4-mile radius.

Item 1a: Distance to Nearest Town. Record the distance from the facility to the city limits of the nearest town or city. If a facility is rural but is located within city limits, answer "0."

Item 2: Type of Neighborhood. To answer this item, consider the area within 1/4 mile of the facility.

Item 3: Number of Buildings. In multiunit facilities, consider only the unit under study when answering this question. For example, if you are assessing a nursing home that occupies one floor of a building in a facility that also has three separate apartment buildings, mark "yes" to indicate that the facility is all in one building.

Sometimes buildings have separate wings or are attached by covered walks or hallways, and it is not clear whether they are one building. In these cases, consider the functioning of the building. If the separation of two structures is bridged in such a way as to allow movement from one unit to the other without changing floors or going outside, consider it to be one building. For example, the structures below are attached in such a way that you do not have to go up or down a flight of stairs to get to the other section; they are functionally a unit.

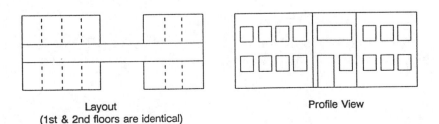

Layout
(1st & 2nd floors are identical)

Profile View

In contrast, the buildings pictured below are functionally separate. If you lived on the second floor in one building and wanted to go to the second floor of the other building, you would have to go down a story, cross over, and then go up a story.

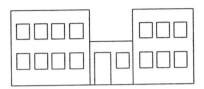

Items 3a, 4a, and 4b: Height of Building. If a building site is sloped so that the building is taller on one side than on the other, answer this question according to functional criteria. If you have to go up half a story or more to enter by the main entrance, count the basement as one story and the first floor as the second story. If the basement is mostly underground, do not count it as a story. If a floor of the building is used only by staff or for utilities, storage, or parking, it should be counted nevertheless, as should an upper floor that only partially covers the floor below.

Item 5: Community Accessibility. Resources that are located on the grounds of the facility, such as a chapel or hospital, should not be considered in answering this question. Count only those resources located in the surrounding community and available to community residents. Once the area within 1/4 mile of the facility is defined, you can drive around it looking for these resources or you can use a local phone book to determine whether these facilities are located within the circle.

Item 7a: Benches. If public transportation does not stop within easy walking distance, mark this item no.

Item 8: Street Lights. To be credited, the street lights should be close enough together to light the entire length of the street and sidewalks.

Section II: Exterior of Building

If one section of a building is being assessed and this unit is on an upper floor, questions about the exterior of the building should be answered for the building as a whole. For example, determine whether the outside walk and entrance are visible from the first floor lobby and from first floor offices.

Item 1: Sheltered Entrance. If an overhang protects a person standing outside the building from sun and from rain, mark yes.

Item 2: Outside Lighting. If it is possible, observe the outside lighting yourself. If this is not possible, ask whether the building is lighted so that there are no shadows or dark areas near traveled pathways or areas frequented by residents.

Item 3: Outside Walk and Entrance Visible. Mark yes if the doorway and portions of the walkway leading to it can be monitored by a person seated in these locations. The office or lobby must be occupied at least some of the time.

Items 4a and 4b: Outside Seating Visible. If there is no outside seating, Items 4a and 4b are "not applicable" (n.a.). If the seats are movable, answer in terms of the locations they actually occupy on your visits to the facility. Mark yes if most of the seating is visible.

Items 4c and 4d: Protected Seating. If there is no outside seating, Items 4c and 4d should be marked no (for the rationale, see Not Applicable Items). If the seats are movable, determine whether they can be placed in a protected location that provides shade on a sunny day and shelter from rain. Mark yes if some of the seating is located in a protected area.

Item 5: Patio or Courtyard. If there is an area that functions as a patio or courtyard, whether it is enclosed or open and whether it is surfaced in concrete or grass, mark yes. If a roof area is appropriately furnished and open to residents, count it as a patio. Do not count the area around the main entrance to the building.

Item 6b: Umbrella Tables. Umbrella tables may be stored during the winter. If you do not see any umbrellas up, ask if they are available and when they are put up. Mark yes if they are put up automatically when warm weather arrives.

Item 6c: Condition of Furniture. Mark yes if the furniture is well maintained, safe, and stable with no splintering, rough edges, and the like.

Item 6d: Covered Area. If the only covered area outside is near the front entrance and has already been credited for Item 4c, mark no.

Item 6e: Sun Screen If the only shaded area outside is near the front entrance and has already been credited for Item 4c, mark no.

Item 7: Garden Area. It may not be apparent whether residents use the garden; ask the administrator or a staff member. Mark yes if the residents have access to garden space.

Item 9: Parking for Handicapped. Mark yes only if spaces for the handicapped are specifically designated as such with signs and special markings.

Item 10: Staff Parking. Mark yes if the facility provides sufficient parking to accommodate all staff. Include on-street parking directly adjacent to the building.

Item 11: Visitor Parking. Mark yes if there are spaces available in addition to those used by staff. If you have difficulty finding parking near the facility, mark no.

Item 12: Acreage. Measure or estimate the acreage yourself or ask a knowledgeable staff member. (One acre = 43,560 square feet or 4,840 square yards.) If you are assessing a multiunit facility, see the directions for prorating (Multiunit Facilities).

Section III, Interior of Building, Part I: Lobby and Entrance Area

Item 2: Number of Entrances. Mark yes if all doors are generally kept locked, if all but one of the doors are generally locked, or if there is only one door, which is left unlocked. For example, if the main entrance is unlocked during the day and staff enter by a separate entrance, which is always locked, mark yes. If the main entrance and staff entrance are both unlocked during the day, mark no.

Item 4: Instructions for Getting in. If the door is never locked, mark yes.

Items 5 and 6: Front Door. If the front door opens and closes automatically mark both items yes. If the door is not automatic and it has to be pulled or pushed closed, mark both items no. If the door is not automatic but swings closed by itself, mark Item 6 yes.

Item 7: Width of Front Door Opening. If the front door opening is at least 3 feet wide, mark yes.

Item 8: Monitoring Access. Answer yes if someone generally observes people as they enter the facility. The individual may be a security guard, a staff member, or a resident assigned this duty. This need not be the individual's only duty, but it must be explicitly assigned. Monitoring need not be 24 hours a day if all doors are locked at night. If the building has more than one unlocked entrance and the main entrance is monitored, answer yes.

Item 9: Reception Desk. Count a nursing station or open office located near the entrance as a reception desk; mark yes only if an employee or resident regularly occupies the reception area or desk.

Item 10: Sign in. If visitors are asked to sign in, mark yes.

Item 11: Lobby. Mark no if the entrance opens directly on a hallway or on an area no wider than the hallway. A lobby is distinguished from a lounge (see Item 13) by its spatial relationship to the entrance. If you walk directly into the area from the outside, it is a lobby. If the room is separated from the entrance area by a visual barrier, such as a planter box or room divider, or by a wall, it is a lounge.

Item 11a: Size of Lobby. Measure the dimensions of the lobby and compute the area at your leisure. If you are assessing one unit of a multiunit building, prorate the lobby area according to the directions under Multiunit Facilities. For example, if three 50-bed units share a building and a single lobby area, the unit under study should be credited with one third of the lobby square footage. If the unit has its own lobby area as well, add this square footage to the prorated area of the main lobby.

Item 13a: Lounge Furnished for Resting. If there is no lounge by the entry, mark this item no.

Item 15: Clock. If a clock is visible from the entrance or the lobby and someone with impaired vision could easily read it, mark yes.

Section III, Part II: Hall and Stairway Areas

Item 1: Hall Width. In some facilities, main hallways vary in width throughout the building. In such cases, measure the main hallways and use the minimum width.

Item 2: Crowded Hallways. If the hallways are crowded with people or objects, mark yes.

Item 4: Hallways Decorated. To be credited, most of the hallways must have some decoration such as plants or pictures.

Item 5b: Accessible Drinking Fountain. If you could drink from the fountain while seated, mark yes. If in doubt, ask a resident in a wheelchair to demonstrate its use. If the fountain is furnished with paper cups that can be filled by someone seated in a wheelchair, mark yes. If there are no fountains, mark Item 5b no.

Item 6: Public Telephones. If there are no public telephones, mark Items 6, 6b, 6c, and 6d no.

Item 6b: Writing Surface. To be credited, at least one telephone on each floor must have a writing surface nearby.

Item 6c: Accessible Telephones. If you could use the phone while seated, mark yes. If the phone is low enough for use from a wheelchair but is blocked by furniture, mark no. If in doubt, have a resident in a wheelchair demonstrate its use.

Item 6d: Loudness Control. Mark yes if the phone has a control to regulate the volume of the caller's voice (not the ring). The volume control is generally located on the receiver.

Item 7: Smoke Detectors. You may have to ask because smoke detectors are not always easily visible. Do not count a heat-activated sprinkler system.

Item 9: Lighting for Stairs. Decide whether the stairs are lighted so that a person with impaired vision would have no trouble seeing the whole stair area. Consider all the stairs within the building and leading to it. If there are no steps in the building, mark this item n.a. If Item 8 is answered no but the facility has some stairs, Item 9 should be answered yes or no as appropriate.

Item 10: Nonskid Surfaces. If there are no stairs or ramps, mark this item n.a.. Consider all the stairs or ramps in the building even if they are not generally used by residents.

Item 11: Color Coding. If the building is only one story (or residents use only one floor) and only one corridor, mark this item yes. To be credited with color coding or numbering of floors, a building must be designed so that people leaving the elevator or stairwell area know immediately what floor they are on. If color coding is used, the colors must be distinctive and each floor or wing must be decorated in a different color. If numbers are used, they must be large and located where they can be readily seen when entering that floor of the building. Small numbers on the apartment doors are not sufficient.

Item 12: Names on Door. Do not credit names on the ends of beds or elsewhere in the room.

Section III, Part III:
Lounge and Community Room Areas

Items 1a, 1b, 1c, and 1d: Lounges. Begin by classifying all the communal areas of the building into one of three categories: lounge, special activity area, or dining room. Use functional criteria. A lounge is an area used mainly for informal activities such as visiting, reading, smoking, and watching TV. A recreation or special activity area is used primarily for more organized or specialized activities such as crafts, movies, discussion groups, or card games. If residents eat in a room but socialize or engage in other informal activities there most of the time, it is a lounge. If they eat in a room but sometimes use it for visiting before and after meals, it is a dining area. Similarly, if organized activities take place in a room but residents use it for informal activities most of the time, it is a lounge. Do not go by the name given to an area but by its actual function. List each communal area in only one category.

If one section of a room is used for one purpose and another section is used for a different purpose, divide the room and give area measurements according to function. For example, the room pictured below is a dining room with a small lounge area.

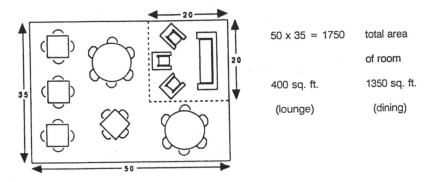

50 x 35 = 1750   total area

of room

400 sq. ft.   1350 sq. ft.

(lounge)   (dining)

When measuring this room, separate the areas as if they were different rooms. In this case, count the 20-foot by 20-foot area as a lounge and the remaining area as a dining area. Tally the lounge area under Section III, Part III and the dining area under Section III, Part V.

You will need to measure all the lounges to complete this section. In multiunit facilities with shared lounge areas, prorate the number and size of lounges according to the example under Multiunit Facilities.

Items 3 and 4: Tables. If tables are suitable for both functions, answer yes to both items. Tables serving these functions may be available in a recreation room or dining room; credit them if residents have free access to them at any time of the day. To count for Item 4, a table must have all four sides accessible or be easy to move.

Item 5: Reading Material. Do not count a library here (it is counted in the next section). If magazines or newspapers are available in a lounge, mark this item yes.

Item 7: Furniture Spacing. The furniture should be spaced to allow 40-inch aisles in all lounges. In addition, there should be areas in which the furniture is 5 feet apart for a wheelchair to turn or for two wheelchairs to pass.

Item 8: Quiet Lounge. To be credited, the lounge must have no television and be out of earshot of a television.

Section III, Part IV:
Recreation or Special Activity Areas

Items 1a, 1b, 1c, and 1d: Special Activity Areas. In determining which rooms are special activity areas, use functional guidelines given in the directions for lounge areas (see Section III, Part I: Lounge and Community Room Areas). To prorate in a multiunit facility, see Multiunit Facilities. Include a library, music room, physical therapy room, craft room, pottery studio, game room, occupational therapy room, auditorium, sewing room, and so on. Do not include a beauty parlor, a laundry room, a gift shop, or medical treatment room. If an area is used for lounging and for occasional activities, such as crafts or movies, it should be counted as a lounge. Count each area only once.

Item 2: Library. This does not have to be a special room. It can be part of a room as long as books can be borrowed. Also count a library cart that is taken around to residents' rooms. Include a separate library room in the square-footage total (Items 1, 1a, b, c, and d).

Item 3: Listening Room. Mark yes only if a room is used primarily for listening to music; include it in the square-footage total (Items 1, 1a, b, c, and d).

Items 5, 8, 9, and 10: Recreational or Activity Materials. This equipment may be stored out of sight. Ask a staff member if it exists. Mark yes only if the equipment is available for use by residents.

Section III, Part V: Dining Room Areas

Make sure that there is no overlap of areas measured; use functional guidelines as described for lounges (see Section III, Part III: Lounge and Community Room Areas). To prorate in a multiunit facility, see Multiunit Facilities.

Item 2, 3, and 4: Dining Tables. Answer these questions even if you have not counted the room in which eating takes place as a dining room because it serves some other principal function. For example, if a lounge has dining tables, note the presence of these tables here. If there is no dining room and residents eat in their own rooms or the halls, answer in terms of the tables available there.

Item 4: Aisle Space. To be credited, spacing of dining room tables should allow wheelchair access to every seating place (i.e., at least 40 inches between all tables and some aisle width of 5 feet to allow two wheelchairs to pass or a wheelchair to turn).

Section III, Part VI: Staff and Office Areas

For Items 1, 2, 3, 4, 6, 7, and 8, credit each office in only one category. The facility need not have a current staff member in a particular role to be credited for having that kind of office space. For example, if there is no social service or counseling staff at the present time, but an office is available for use by such a person, credit the facility with that office space.

Item 5: Distractions. Stand inside the office. If you think you would be distracted if you were working there, mark no.

Item 8: Staff Lounge. Do not count a resident lounge used by staff. To be credited, an area must be designated as the staff lounge. If there is no staff lounge, mark Items 8a and 8b no.

Item 9: Staff Members. If you are also completing the Resident and Staff Information Form (RESIF), complete RESIF Section III: Part I and add up the staff full-time equivalent (FTE) hours in each position to obtain the total number of staff members (FTEs). If you are not completing the RESIF, use payroll sheets or other records showing the number of hours staff work in a given period. To calculate FTEs, divide the number of hours worked in a week by 40. If this information is not available, ask the administrator to estimate the number of full-time-equivalent employees and use this information to complete this item. All staff, not just those providing resident care, should be included.

Section III, Part VII: General Facilities

Item 1: Map of Resources. This refers to a map showing the surrounding neighborhood and its resources, not a map of the facility itself.

Items 3a and 4a: Pictures. If pictures of residents are posted by their door along with their name or if staff pictures with names are posted on a bulletin board, mark these items yes.

Items 5, 6, 9, 11, and 12. These areas or features are sometimes difficult to find. Ask to see them, and find out if the residents are allowed to use them.

Section III, Part VIII: Bathroom and Toilet Areas.

If there are separate shower rooms or bathing areas, as is often the case in nursing homes, Questions 1 through 9 apply equally to these areas.

Item 1: Raised Threshold. A raised threshold is any variation in the level of the floor such as a metal strip.

Item 2: Doors Open out. If there are toilet stalls, this question applies to the doors to the stalls.

Item 7: Nonslip Surfaces. Mark yes if there are obvious strips of sand-paper-like material glued over the tiles to prevent slipping.

Items 10 and 11: Size of Bathrooms. Do not include shower rooms or bathing areas in nursing homes when determining the size of the largest and smallest bathrooms. Measure areas that contain the toilet and sink. Indicate the sizes of the largest and smallest bathrooms for the entire facility.

Items 13a and 13b: Bathtubs and Showers. If the tub and shower are together in one fixture they should be counted in both categories.

Item 13c: Flexible Shower. Mark yes if the shower has a long hose that can be directed at any part of the body.

Section III, Part IX:
Individual Rooms or Apartments

Items 1, 2, and 3: Number of Rooms and Number of Residents. If you are also completing the Policy and Program Information Form, this information can be obtained from Sections I and II. If not, you may need to ask about these items. Count only those rooms or apartments actually occupied at the present time.

Item 4: Wall Space for Pictures. Visit a number of resident rooms to determine whether the facility allows residents to display pictures on the walls.

Item 5: Wall or Table Lamps. If there are wall or table lamps that provide enough light for reading, even for the visually impaired, mark yes.

Item 7: Window Sill. The window sill should be at least 6 inches wide.

Items 8 and 9: Floors and Walls. These questions refer to light colors, not bright ones (i.e., yellow is light, orange is usually not).

Items 10 and 11: Heating and Air-Conditioning Controls. You may have to ask because these controls are not always easily visible. If there is no air conditioning, Item 11 should be marked very few or none.

Item 13: Room for Wheelchairs. Determine whether pieces of furniture are at least 40 inches apart and whether the room has a space with a 5-foot radius for a wheelchair to turn around.

Item 15: Smoke Detectors. You may have to ask whether there are smoke detectors in the individual rooms or apartments. Do not count a sprinkler system.

Item 16: Call Button. If the facility is divided into rooms, each room must have a call button or telephone for "all" to be an appropriate response. For apartments, each studio apartment and all bedrooms must have a call button or telephone to be credited.

Item 17: Kitchen. This item is n.a. in facilities that do not have apartments.

Items 20 and 21: Closets. Measure all the closet areas in the room or bedrooms and divide the area by the number of people using them. Do not count living room, kitchen, or bathroom cabinets or closets in these totals.

5

POLICY AND PROGRAM
INFORMATION FORM

The Policy and Program Information Form (POLIF) measures the policies and services of group residential settings for older people. It comprises 130 scored items that focus on facility policies, the types of rooms available, how the facility is organized, and what services are provided. Additional items provide descriptive information about admission fees, facility management, and the use of services. Information is obtained from interviews with administrators and other staff.

The POLIF measures the actual facility. We have also adapted the POLIF to assess individuals' preferences about facility policies and services (POLIF Form I).

POLIF SUBSCALES

The nine POLIF subscales are presented in Table 5.1. The first two subscales reflect the extent to which behavioral requirements are imposed on residents. The Expectations for Functioning subscale measures the minimum standards for self-care, and the Acceptance of Problem Behavior subscale assesses the extent to which uncooperative, aggressive, or eccentric behavior is accepted in the facility.

The second set of POLIF subscales measures the balance between individual freedom and institutional order and stability. The four areas cover the degree to which residents have the option of establishing their

TABLE 5.1 Policy and Program Information Form (POLIF) Subscale
Descriptions

Subscale	*Description*
	Behavioral requirements for residents
Expectations for Functioning	Minimum capacity to perform daily living functions that is acceptable in the facility
Acceptance of Problem Behavior	Extent to which aggressive, defiant, destructive, or eccentric behavior is tolerated
	Individual freedom and institutional order
Policy Choice	Extent to which the facility allows residents to individualize their routines
Resident Control	How much residents are involved in facility administration and influence facility policies
Policy Clarity	Extent of formal institutional mechanisms for defining expected behavior and communicating ideas
Provision for Privacy	The amount of privacy given to residents
	Provision of services and activities
Availability of Health Services	The availability of health services in the facility
Availability of Daily Living Assistance	The availability of facility services that assist residents in tasks of daily living
Availability of Social-Recreational Activities	The availability of organized activities within the facility

own daily routines (Policy Choice), the presence of formal institutional structures that provide residents with potential influence in the facility (Resident Control) and that offer opportunities to communicate about the policies and programs (Policy Clarity), and the amount of privacy available to residents (Provision for Privacy).

The third set of POLIF subscales measures the availability of services and activities. The subscales tap the provision of health services, daily living assistance, and social-recreational activities. We also included questions about the use of these services, which can help describe the resident population or provide an index of program outcomes. Normative data and the scoring key for these three service utilization dimensions are presented in Appendix E.

NORMATIVE SAMPLES AND
PSYCHOMETRIC CHARACTERISTICS

Normative Samples

Normative data for the POLIF are available from two samples of facilities for older adults: 262 community facilities and 81 facilities serving veterans (see Normative Samples in Chapter 1).

Most items on the POLIF are scored dichotomously to indicate the presence or absence of particular policies or services. The exception is Availability of Social-Recreational Activities; here, activities are weighted according to their frequency. For items that are not presented in a dichotomous format, we developed dichotomous scoring criteria based on conceptual criteria and the actual distributions obtained in our sample of facilities.

The raw scores for a facility are percentage scores reflecting the number of policies or services offered out of the total number possible. For example, Acceptance of Problem Behavior asks about policies regarding 16 problem behaviors. Facility scores can vary from 0% to 100%. A facility that has 8 of the 16 items in the direction of greater tolerance obtains a raw score of 50%. The average score for the total community sample on Acceptance of Problem Behavior is 46%. Each of the means and standard deviations in Table 5.2 was derived in a similar way.

The POLIF itself is in Appendix A, hand-scoring worksheets are in Appendix B, and directions for converting raw percentage scores to standard scores are in Appendix C.

Community Facilities

Means and standard deviations for the nine POLIF subscales for the total community sample and for each of the three subsamples are reported in Table 5.2. The sample of community facilities varied considerably on all nine subscales as shown by the standard deviations in Table 5.2.

The norms for the three types of community facilities reflect meaningful variations among types of residential settings. For example, apartments are highest, residential care facilities are intermediate, and nursing homes are lowest on three subscales: Expectations for Functioning, Policy Choice, and Provision for Privacy. Apartments are also higher than nursing homes on Resident Control. The pattern is reversed on the three subscales tapping the provision of services and activities: Nursing homes

TABLE 5.2 POLIF Subscale Means and Standard Deviations for the Total
Community Sample and the Three Subsamples

Subscale	Total Sample (n = 262 Facilities)		Nursing Homes (n = 135 Facilities)		Residential Care (n = 60 Facilities)		Apartments (n = 67 Facilities)	
	Mean	SD	Mean	SD	Mean	SD	Mean	SD
Expectations for Functioning	35	33	11	16	42	24	78	16
Acceptance of Problem Behavior	46	22	47	23	39	23	50	16
Policy Choice	55	24	43	17	51	22	84	9
Resident Control	36	19	31	16	35	21	49	17
Policy Clarity	63	21	69	16	55	26	58	23
Provision for Privacy	54	30	34	14	56	27	93	7
Availability of Health Services	46	28	65	14	41	25	13	16
Availability of Daily Living Assistance	70	27	87	9	76	14	32	19
Availability of Social-Recreational Activities	62	22	73	15	54	26	47	19

provide more health services, help residents more in their daily activities,
and provide more organized activities than do apartments. Residential
care facilities are intermediate on the availability of health services and
daily living assistance and similar to apartments in the number of
organized activities. Residential care facilities score lower than apartments on Acceptance of Problem Behavior, and nursing homes are
highest on Policy Clarity.

Veterans Facilities

The POLIF means and standard deviations for the sample of 81
veterans facilities and for each of the two subsamples are given in Table 5.3.
Most of the subscales discriminate both between the two subsamples and
among facilities of each type. Compared with domiciliaries, veterans
nursing care units have fewer behavioral requirements for residents

TABLE 5.3 POLIF Subscale Means and Standard Deviations for the Total
Veterans Sample and the Two Subsamples

Subscale	Total Sample (n = 81 Facilities)		Nursing Care Units (n = 57 Facilities)		Domiciliaries (n = 24 Facilities)	
	Mean	SD	Mean	SD	Mean	SD
Expectations for Functioning	28	32	11	16	69	24
Acceptance of Problem Behavior	50	23	54	22	40	24
Policy Choice	37	17	35	16	42	21
Resident Control	28	17	23	15	38	15
Policy Clarity	76	16	72	16	86	11
Provision for Privacy	33	20	28	14	46	26
Availability of Health Services	93	12	96	7	86	17
Availability of Daily Living Assistance	89	13	94	8	79	16
Availability of Social-Recreational Activities	63	17	63	17	61	19

(lower expectations for functioning and greater acceptance of problem
behavior) and provide more health and daily living assistance services.
Domiciliaries give residents more control, have clearer policies, and
provide more privacy.

Compared with the community normative sample, the veterans facilities tend to provide more services and to impose more structure on
residents' lives. The veterans nursing care units provide more health and
personal care services than do community nursing homes, but they have
lower levels of resident choice, control, and privacy and fewer organized
activities. Compared with residential care facilities, domiciliaries have
higher expectations for functioning, place more emphasis on policy
clarity, and provide more health services, but they have less privacy.

Subscale Internal Consistencies
and Intercorrelations

Table 5.4 shows the number of items on each of the POLIF subscales
and provides estimates of internal consistency (Cronbach's alpha). The

TABLE 5.4 POLIF Subscale Internal Consistency and Test-Retest Reliability

Subscale	Number of Items	Internal Consistency	Test-Retest Reliability (n = 12 Facilities)
Expectations for Functioning	11	.88	.81
Acceptance of Problem Behavior	16	.79	.72
Policy Choice	19	.76	.96
Resident Control	29	.80	.84
Policy Clarity	10	.69	.79
Provision for Privacy	10	.83	.95
Availability of Health Services	8	.73	.90
Availability of Daily Living Assistance	14	.89	.92
Availability of Social-Recreational Activities	13	.79	.81

alphas are based on data from more than 140 facilities in the community sample. The internal consistencies are quite high for eight of the subscales and moderate for the remaining one, Policy Clarity.

The intercorrelations among the nine subscales (partial correlations controlling for level of care) for the community sample are shown above the diagonal in Table 5.5. The subscale intercorrelations are relatively low (average $r = .20$), with the exception of moderate relationships among Policy Choice, Resident Control, and Provision for Privacy. As expected, facilities that give residents more privacy also allow them more choice and control. In general, however, the nine subscales measure reasonably distinct aspects of a facility's policy and service resources. The intercorrelations for veterans facilities are shown below the diagonal in Table 5.5; they provide additional support for the conclusion that the subscales tap somewhat distinct aspects of a facility's organizational environment.

Interobserver Reliability, Test-Retest Reliability, and Profile Stability

To obtain interobserver reliability data for the POLIF, the project observer, two staff members, and three residents independently completed the POLIF in 15 facilities. We found that facility residents and

TABLE 5.5 Partial Correlations Among POLIF Subscales, With Level of Care Controlled[a]

Subscale	Expectations for Functioning	Acceptance of Problem Behavior	Policy Choice	Resident Control	Policy Clarity	Provision for Privacy	Availability of Health Services	Availability of Daily Living Assistance	Availability of Social-Recreational Activities
Expectations for Functioning	—	.09	.16	.20	.17	.11	.08	-.14	-.02
Acceptance of Problem Behavior	-.16	—	.32	.27	.06	.13	.10	-.02	.08
Policy Choice	.14	.12	—	.48	.26	.52	.08	-.07	.21
Resident Control	.07	.03	.44	—	.38	.44	.22	.09	.22
Policy Clarity	.06	-.11	.18	.32	—	.24	.31	.21	.33
Provision for Privacy	-.01	-.10	.37	.41	.17	—	.13	-.07	.21
Availability of Health Services	-.12	.00	.17	.30	.08	.00	—	.34	.24
Availability of Daily Living Assistance	-.20	-.06	-.07	.18	.06	.34	.07	—	.18
Availability of Social-Recreational Activities	.11	.02	.29	.53	.32	.19	.16	.22	—

a. Correlations above the diagonal are for the community sample; correlations below the diagonal are for the veterans sample.

staff members can serve as alternate or additional sources of information and that reliability is improved substantially when the responses from two or three individuals are pooled. Perhaps surprisingly, residents agree somewhat more closely with the administrator than do staff members. Residents show substantially higher agreement with the administrator than do staff in rating availability of health services and daily living assistance. In rating acceptance of problem behavior, however, residents and staff fail to reach consensus with the administrator or with one another.

Subscale and profile stability data were obtained by readministering the POLIF in 12 of these facilities after an interval of 9 to 12 months. The test-retest results, shown in Table 5.4, indicate that the subscales have moderate to high test-retest reliability. The profile stability for each of the 12 facilities was computed by calculating intraclass correlations on the POLIF standard scores for the two administrations in the facility. These correlations ranged from .62 to .98; 9 of the 12 correlations were above .80.

THE IDEAL FORM

The Ideal Form of the POLIF (POLIF Form I) measures individuals' preferences regarding policies and services of group residential facilities. Form I has 130 items, each of which is parallel to an item on the POLIF.

Development

We developed the POLIF Form I by rewording POLIF items to elicit information about individual preferences. Thus, for example, the POLIF item "Does the facility have an orientation program for new residents?" was reworded as "Should there be an orientation program for new residents?" We tried to keep the individual items as simple as possible and, to facilitate administration of Form I in either a written questionnaire or interview format, worded all items as questions.

The items on five of the nine subscales are answered on a 4-point scale varying from "not important" to "desirable," "very important," and "essential." The four other subscales (Expectations for Functioning, Acceptance of Problem Behavior, Policy Choice, and Resident Control) pertain to policies that some may view as undesirable; these items are answered on a 4-point scale ranging from "definitely not" to "preferably not," "preferably yes," and "definitely yes." After a series of item trials and revisions, we constructed a version of the POLIF Form I composed of all nine POLIF subscales (for more details, see Brennan, Moos, & Lemke, 1989). The POLIF Form I was administered to the same nine groups of respondents that completed the Physical and Architectural Features Checklist (PAF) Form I (see Development in Chapter 4).

Because the POLIF Form I helps people describe the type of facility they would like, it can facilitate comparisons of the preferences of administrators, staff, residents, potential residents, and experts. It can also reveal individual variations in preferences, which should be considered when planning residential settings for heterogeneous groups of older people. Used with the POLIF, Form I helps to measure person-environment congruence by contrasting the preferences of current or potential residents with the actual qualities of a setting. It can thus identify areas in which respondents want change. (For further details on potential applications, see Brennan et al., 1989; Moos, Lemke, & Clayton, 1983; Moos, Lemke, & David, 1987.)

The POLIF Form I and scoring directions are provided in Appendix D.

Normative Samples

The means and standard deviations of POLIF Form I subscales are shown in Table 5.6 for residents, Table 5.7 for staff, and Table 5.8 for potential residents and experts. The scores are given in terms of the average percentage of items rated preferably yes or definitely yes (for the first four dimensions) or very important or essential (for the last five dimensions) by the average respondent. A 4-point scoring system (varying from 0 for not important or definitely not to 3 for essential or definitely yes) results in roughly comparable percentage means and standard deviations; investigators who wish to use a 4-point scoring system can compare their results with the means and standard deviations shown in Appendix D.

Using dichotomous scoring, an individual who rates 8 of the 16 Acceptance of Problem Behavior items as preferably yes or definitely yes obtains a score of 50%. The average endorsement rate on Acceptance of Problem Behavior was 11% for the 422 residents, 21% for staff, and 38% for experts as shown in Tables 5.6, 5.7, and 5.8. Each of the means and standard deviations in Tables 5.6, 5.7, and 5.8 was derived in the same way. The standard deviations indicate substantial individual differences in preferences for policy and program factors in all groups of respondents.

TABLE 5.6 POLIF Form I Subscale Means and Standard Deviations for the
Total Sample and the Three Subsamples of Residents

Subscale	Total Sample of Residents (n = 422)		Nursing Home Residents (n = 40)		Residential Care Residents (n = 153)		Apartment Residents (n = 229)	
	Mean	SD	Mean	SD	Mean	SD	Mean	SD
Expectations for Functioning	68	28	18	21	65	25	77	22
Acceptance of Problem Behavior	11	17	26	27	12	19	9	12
Policy Choice	72	18	52	16	65	18	79	15
Resident Control	62	23	44	21	73	20	57	21
Policy Clarity	50	32	51	25	60	32	43	30
Provision for Privacy	68	28	42	24	57	31	79	20
Availability of Health Services	40	38	59	26	63	37	22	29
Availability of Daily Living Assistance	32	27	61	19	38	30	24	22
Availability of Social-Recreational Activities	32	32	51	29	38	35	26	28

Importance of Policies and Services

Overall, residents desire high standards for resident functioning and
conformity to behavioral norms. As expected, most older people want
to regulate their own daily activities and to have some influence on
facility policies. Specifically, a majority of the individuals in each group
want to be able to choose when to wake up, when to take a bath or
shower, where to sit at meals, and when to go to bed. They also want to
have house meetings, committees that include residents as members, and
a residents' council that meets regularly. On the other hand, a majority
of respondents feel that residents should not be involved in personnel
matters, selection of residents, or decisions about when a resident should
be moved.

Among the services, residents rate health services as more important
overall than organized recreational activities and assistance with tasks
of daily living. This ranking of services is somewhat surprising given
that inability to perform activities of daily living often precipitates the

TABLE 5.7 POLIF Form I Subscale Means and Standard Deviations for the Total Sample and the Three Subsamples of Staff

Subscale	Total Sample of Staff (n = 98) Mean SD		Nursing Home Staff (n = 33) Mean SD		Residential Care Staff (n = 34) Mean SD		Apartment Staff (n = 31) Mean SD	
Expectations for Functioning	54	34	17	23	63	20	82	20
Acceptance of Problem Behavior	21	24	23	22	9	14	30	30
Policy Choice	70	21	59	25	72	17	80	15
Resident Control	56	20	56	22	53	19	60	17
Policy Clarity	62	25	67	25	55	27	63	23
Provision for Privacy	67	29	44	26	71	27	86	13
Availability of Health Services	45	34	74	18	36	31	24	29
Availability of Daily Living Assistance	54	32	76	27	57	24	27	23
Availability of Social-Recreational Activities	65	35	83	29	59	34	53	36

move to a congregate setting. It may reflect older people's belief that good health (as a result of good medical care) is the best assurance of functional independence. Of the health services, residents feel most strongly about regularly scheduled doctor's and nurse's hours, having a doctor on call, and being able to obtain assistance in the use of prescribed medications.

A majority of residents want to have at least one meal served each day, with almost a third of the residents strongly desiring all three meals. A transportation service, which can link residents to a variety of resources in the community, is also seen as very important. Substantial minorities also value a barber or beauty service and assistance with housekeeping and cleaning, laundry, shopping, and financial matters. The organized activities that are most often preferred include exercise or physical fitness groups, arts and crafts, religious services, organized games such as bingo, and classes and discussion groups.

TABLE 5.8 POLIF Form I Subscale Means and Standard Deviations for Potential Residents and Experts

Subscale	Potential Nursing Home Residents (n = 30)		Potential Apartment Residents (n = 205)		Experts Describing Apartments (n = 44)	
	Mean	SD	Mean	SD	Mean	SD
Expectations for Functioning	45	36	60	28	47	23
Acceptance of Problem Behavior	9	16	10	14	38	26
Policy Choice	69	17	78	18	96	7
Resident Control	60	19	73	22	90	11
Policy Clarity	57	27	53	31	75	22
Provision for Privacy	63	22	69	26	89	14
Availability of Health Services	50	36	45	36	57	29
Availability of Daily Living Assistance	35	32	29	26	56	25
Availability of Social-Recreational Activities	28	30	31	31	59	28

Differences Among Resident and Staff Groups

The data show substantial differences among residents of the three types of facilities on several Form I subscales. As expected, apartment residents prefer much higher expectations for functioning, policy choice, and privacy and much lower service and activity availability than do residential care facility residents. Nursing home residents score lowest of any resident group on Expectations for Functioning, Policy Choice, Resident Control, and Provision for Privacy; they score highest on Acceptance of Problem Behavior and on Availability of Daily Living Assistance and Social-Recreational Activities. Formal provision for resident involvement and clear communication is most salient for residential care residents who may feel constrained by their residential setting yet function well enough to want greater involvement.

Apartment residents asked to rate an ideal nursing home (Table 5.8) respond like apartment residents rating an apartment in terms of their tolerance for problem behavior and their preferences for resident control and for activities (Table 5.6). Their scores on Expectations for Functioning, Policy Choice, Provision for Privacy, Availability of Health Services, and Availability of Daily Living Assistance are midway between those of apartment and nursing home residents. In general, older people in their own homes (Table 5.8) see the ideal apartment in much the same way as do current apartment residents (Table 5.6), but they value resident control and availability of health services more highly.

As shown in Table 5.7, differences among staff parallel differences among residents in the three types of facilities. Staff in nursing homes rate services much more important and expectations about functioning, flexibility, and privacy lower than do staff of apartments. Compared with staff working in apartments, experts prefer more emphasis in several of the areas—most notably, policy choice, resident control, and policy clarity (Tables 5.7 and 5.8). In addition, experts are more likely to endorse lower expectations for functioning and more provision of supportive services.

Subscale Internal Consistencies and Intercorrelations

The POLIF Form I subscale internal consistencies (Cronbach's alpha) were calculated on the overall sample of 799 respondents; all are relatively high ($r = .81$ or higher). The intercorrelations among the eight POLIF Form I subscales (partial correlations controlling for the type of facility) are low to moderate for residents, staff members, and experts. There are moderately strong positive relationships between the three availability dimensions and between these dimensions and Policy Clarity. Most of the subscale correlations, however, are quite low. Individuals' preferences for policy and service resources vary considerably among subscales.

USING THE POLIF TO DESCRIBE GROUP RESIDENCES

The POLIF has been used widely in characterizing facilities and evaluating programs. It helps to describe facilities, to monitor program changes over time, and to promote program improvement. When Form R and Form I are both used, they can alert administrators to discrepancies between a facility's features and resident or staff preferences. When the POLIF is used with other Multiphase Environmental Assessment Proce-

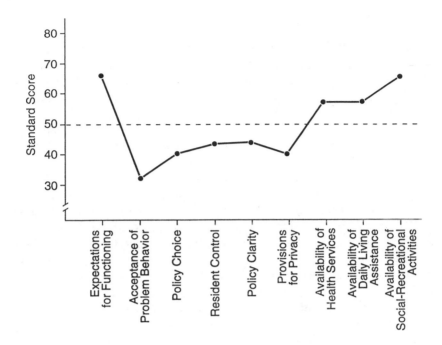

Figure 5.1. POLIF Profile for City Haven Nursing Home

dure (MEAP) instruments, it can help characterize the quality of a residential setting. Chapters 1 and 8 describe in detail the applications of the MEAP.

Profile Interpretation

The POLIF can be used to provide a systematic description of the policies and services in a facility. The POLIF is most useful for such formative evaluations when results are expressed in terms of the conditions that generally prevail in the appropriate normative sample.

To illustrate the interpretation of facility profiles, we present POLIF profiles of the three facilities introduced in Chapter 2. Results are shown as standard scores (based on the appropriate normative sample) with a mean of 50 and a standard deviation of 10. (For additional examples of POLIF profiles, see Lemke & Moos, 1985; Moos & Lemke, 1994; Moos et al., 1987.)

City Haven Nursing Home

Figure 5.1 shows the POLIF profile for City Haven Nursing Home, an average-sized, urban nursing facility. City Haven has a rather typical resident population, except that residents are rather inactive. It offers good community access and ample staff facilities but relatively few other physical resources.

Compared with policies in community nursing homes, residents in City Haven are expected to function more independently and to conform more to socially acceptable behavior (high Expectations for Functioning and low Acceptance of Problem Behavior). City Haven offers fewer opportunities than do most nursing homes in our sample for residents to make choices, exert control over policies, and enjoy privacy. Despite these restrictions on resident behavior, there are relatively few mechanisms for communicating expectations to residents and staff (low Policy Clarity). In contrast with the somewhat restrictive policies, City Haven offers ample program resources. It offers a variety of health care services and daily living assistance. Because of cooperation with a community agency, a rich program of social and recreational activities is available, including discussion groups, meditation, and adult education classes, as well as the more typical nursing home activities.

El Dorado Residential Care Facility

El Dorado is a west coast facility run by a nonprofit corporation. As the residential care section of a continuing care home, it serves an older, mainly female population with above-average independence in daily activities. This older building in a suburban community provides a comfortable and stimulating environment, but one with limited prosthetic features.

Consistent with the high level of functioning shown by residents, the policies require residents to maintain independence in daily activities (see Figure 5.2). Some degree of mental confusion or depression is accepted, but a reduction in independence would lead to pressure to move into the nursing unit. Policies concerning problem behavior are similar to those established by most residential care facilities.

The policies with respect to resident choice and provisions for communicating policies to residents and staff are typical, as is the level of resident control. Residents can get up, bathe, and go to bed whenever they wish, but meals are served at a set time. Monthly house meetings are held, and residents are consulted about menus, residents' complaints,

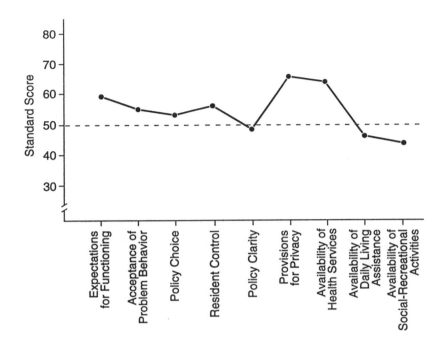

Figure 5.2. POLIF Profile for El Dorado Residential Care Facility

and moving residents within the facility. On the other hand, El Dorado does not have a residents' council, and residents have little voice in areas such as planning activities, dealing with safety concerns, or personnel retention. It has no formal arrangements for orienting new residents, but staff members are given a handbook and orientation and meet regularly. El Dorado offers residents a high level of privacy: Each resident has a private room and bathroom and an individual mailbox, and residents are permitted to close and lock their doors.

The presence of a nursing unit allows El Dorado to offer residents many more health services than do most residential care facilities. There are regularly scheduled physicians' and nurses' hours as well as physical therapy and assistance in using prescribed medications. The high level of supportive services does not extend to daily living assistance, which is about average, consistent with the stated policies and the actual functional abilities of residents. The formal activity program offers only the most commonly provided activities.

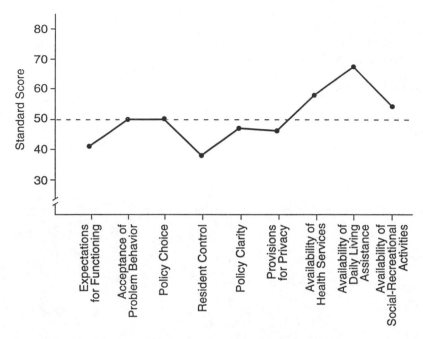

Figure 5.3. POLIF Profile for Marlborough Arms Apartments

Marlborough Arms Apartments

Marlborough Arms is run by a proprietary corporation that also administers a number of other facilities in the northwest. Marlborough Arms serves a somewhat older, more impaired population than do most apartments. As shown by the PAF profile, the physical environment is fairly typical of senior apartments, except that it offers much more space.

The policies, which permit somewhat more impairment than is usually found in apartments, are consistent with the characteristics of the resident population (Figure 5.3). Residents are not expected to clean their own apartments, and some confusion or disorientation is accepted. On the other hand, the policies regarding problem behavior are typical of apartments.

Although residents are given an average level of choice in determining their daily routine, they are offered few formal opportunities for influencing decisions. There is a monthly house meeting, but there are no residents' committees or council and residents have little influence on the activity program, decor of public areas, or handling of residents' complaints. The procedures for communicating policies to staff and residents and the opportunities for privacy are fairly typical of apartments.

In addition to having policies that allow the admission of a somewhat more impaired population, Marlborough Arms supports these individuals with a program that provides more health services and much more assistance with daily living than is usual for apartments. Staff can assist residents with prescribed medications, and a staff member is qualified to provide personal counseling. In addition to providing three meals a day, Marlborough Arms offers housekeeping, assistance with personal care, laundry service, assistance with shopping, and transportation. As in most apartments, the activity program emphasizes organized activities that have broad appeal.

Comparing Actual and Preferred Policies and Services

Information about preferences can help in identifying problems and planning interventions, matching residents with facilities, and understanding the perspectives of different interest groups such as facility staff and residents.

Preferences of Apartment Residents

To illustrate these ideas, we compare the actual features of Marlborough Arms with a description of the ideal congregate apartment. The ideal profile presented in Figure 5.4 is based on POLIF Form I responses of the normative group of congregate apartment residents (also shown in Table 5.6). Similar comparisons can be made with the preferences of an individual respondent such as a current or prospective resident. In Figure 5.4, each real and ideal subscale score is presented as a percentage score. The open bar represents the actual environment of Marlborough Arms, and the darkened area represents the preferences of apartment residents.

Marlborough Arms meets average preferences in all but three areas tapped by the POLIF; residents want substantially less acceptance of problem behavior, higher expectations for functioning, and more resident control of policies than Marlborough Arms provides. In addition, Marlborough Arms offers more daily living services and organized activities than apartment residents view as necessary.

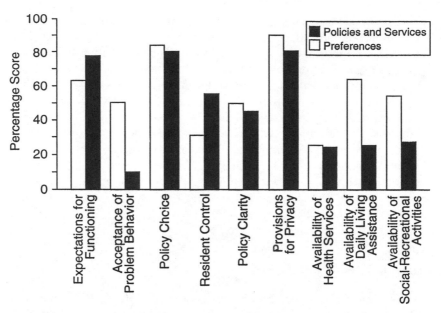

Figure 5.4. Policies and Services in Marlborough Arms and Preferences of Apartment Residents

Another way to compare real and ideal policies and services is to determine whether a facility's policies are consistent with the majority opinion of a particular target group (for items that can be endorsed or rejected) and whether the facility provides the specific resources that are rated very important by a given percentage of respondents. For example, one might determine that if at least 25% of respondents rate an item very important, it should be considered a key resource.

Such a comparison shows that Marlborough Arms generally fulfills apartment residents' preferences. Management policies coincide with the majority opinion of apartment residents for 8 of the 11 items regarding expectations for functioning and for 18 of the 19 items regarding policy choice. In contrast, the policies are less consistent with preferences in the area of acceptance of problem behavior and resident control. Although the facility will accept the presence of residents who refuse to participate in activities, refuse to take prescribed medications, wander around the building or grounds at night, or create a disturbance, most congregate apartment residents believe these behaviors should not be tolerated. A majority of respondents think that residents should be involved in chores around the facility, serve on committees, help produce a newsletter, and have a residents' council, which are all opportunities that are not available to them.

Marlborough Arms matches the residents' overall preferences on policy clarity, but a significant minority (25%-50%) think it is important to have an orientation handbook and a regular newsletter, which are resources Marlborough Arms does not provide. Few health services are available at Marlborough Arms, consistent with the overall preferences of apartment residents. Here again, some residents would like to have regular nurse's hours and an on-call doctor. Marlborough Arms provides transportation, assistance with shopping, a barber-beauty service, and dinner 5 days a week; these are the daily living services rated most important by apartment residents. Similarly, the organized activities are well matched to the priorities established by congregate apartment residents. Almost all activities preferred by at least 25% of congregate apartment residents are actually available.

ADMINISTRATION OF THE POLIF

General Directions for the POLIF

To complete the POLIF, which includes questions about administrative policy and organizational structure, you will need the administrator's assistance for approximately 1 hour. If the administrator is not available, a knowledgeable staff member can substitute, as detailed under Alternate Sources of Information. You may also need to tabulate information from records of service use or from staff members. Review the POLIF with the administrator to determine the best sources of information for each section.

Chapter 2 provides suggestions for presenting the MEAP to facility administrators and staff, setting policies about confidentiality and the use of results, and encouraging cooperation in the data collection process.

Multiunit Facilities

In multiunit facilities, you will need to clearly define the unit you want to study before starting data collection (see Defining the Unit in Chapter 2). Be sure that policies and services are uniform within that unit and that the administrator and other staff members respond to questions in terms of the unit under study.

Not Applicable Items

All items apply to all facilities except where specifically noted under the directions for individual questions. The following examples illustrate the rationale used to determine whether an item can be considered "not applicable." For most items, their presence is an asset and their absence is a liability that detracts from a characteristic of the organizational environment. For example, the Resident Control subscale includes the question "Does the residents' council meet twice a month or more often?" This item is applicable in all cases whether or not there is a residents' council. If there is no residents' council at all (or if the council meets less often than twice a month), this item should be marked "no." A residents' council that meets twice monthly or more often is a potential resource for increasing residents' involvement and can be provided in any type of facility. The absence of a weekly or biweekly residents' council diminishes the opportunities for resident input.

In contrast, items that can be considered not applicable contribute to an aspect of the organizational environment, but their absence does not detract from it. For example, the item "Can residents choose to sit wherever they want at meals?" is not applicable in facilities in which meals are not provided, because the issue of policy choice (freedom to choose where to sit during meals) does not arise if no meals are served.

Alternate Sources of Information

For most dimensions, residents or staff members can serve as alternative sources of information if the administrator is not available. Averaging the independent responses of two or three individuals will substantially improve reliability. Interviewing the respondent ensures uniform interpretation of questions, whereas having staff members use written directions to complete the POLIF has good, although somewhat lower, reliability. Because our data indicate that staff and residents do not agree with each other or with the administrator on the Acceptance of Problem Behavior subscale, we recommend obtaining this information from the administrator.

Scoring

Hand scoring can be accomplished using the reproducible worksheets in Appendix B. Appendix C contains tables for transforming raw percentage scores into standard scores. Allow 1 1/2 hours to score and profile the POLIF.

Directions for the POLIF Form I

Chapter 2 contains detailed suggestions for administering the POLIF Form I to facility residents and staff. The POLIF Form I and its scoring instructions are available in Appendix D.

Specific Directions for the POLIF

Section I: Financial and Entrance Arrangements

Item 1: Minimum Entrance Fee. Check the category that includes the minimum fee required to enter the facility. This does not include a security deposit or payment in advance for a month's rent.

Item 2: Minimum Monthly Rate. Answer this question if any residents pay a set monthly fee. Check the category that includes the lowest monthly fee that residents pay if they are not receiving any government assistance, rate reductions, or Medicaid contributions. If a per diem rate is given, calculate the monthly rate on a 30-day month. If no residents pay a set fee, check the box labeled "less than $200."

Item 7: Capacity. This question asks how many residents could live in the facility if it were completely full. In licensed facilities, this is the number of residents the facility is licensed to care for. In apartments, assume that the facility has maximum occupancy when two people live in each one- or two-bedroom apartment and one person lives in each studio apartment.

Section II: Types of Rooms and Features Available

Although the administrator will often have records of the available types of rooms and features, because of vacancies you may need to count the number of bedrooms, baths, or apartments in the different categories. A floor plan that indicates who lives in each room or a list of residents with their room numbers is helpful. You may have to walk through the facility, count the occupied beds in each room, and determine which bathrooms are shared.

Items 1a, 1b, 1c, 1d, and 1e: Division Into Rooms. Answer these questions in terms of current conditions in the facility—for example, the number of residents now in double rooms. If a room is not occupied, do not count it in these totals. Classify as rooms (rather than as apartments) any individual units that do not contain a kitchen or kitchenette, such as single-room occupancy hotels, and suites of rooms that open on a common area such as a living room and kitchen.

Items 1g, 1h, 1i, and 1j: Bathrooms. Do not count shared shower rooms or bathing areas in nursing homes or other facilities. Count areas used for residents' regular toileting needs.

Item 2a: Number of Apartments. Count only the number of apartments occupied at the present time.

Item 3c: Dressers. If all rooms are unfurnished, mark "yes."

Section III, Organizational Policies, Part I:
General Information

Items 5 and 6: Handbook. Ask to see the handbook given to new residents or staff. Credit the handbook only if it contains fairly complete information about services, rules, and procedures; a brochure describing the facility is not sufficient.

Items 7 and 8: Orientation Program. To be credited, the orientation program must be a formal and systematic procedure for introducing the new resident or staff member to the facility and its procedures.

Item 9a: Frequency of Staff Meetings. Different staff groups may meet with different frequency. For example, department heads may meet once a week and nursing staff may meet once a month. Credit the facility with the most frequent formal staff meeting. Do not count informal discussions among staff such as those that may occur when there is a change in shift.

Section III, Part II: Rules Related to
Personal Possessions and Behaviors

Items 1 and 7: Liquor. Because alcohol is classified as a drug for certain purposes (especially in nursing homes), staff may need to obtain a doctor's permission before they allow residents to drink alcohol. In such cases, "encouraged" would imply that the facility staff set up situations in which drinking alcohol takes place and that staff actively seek permission from physicians for residents to drink. "Allowed" implies that the staff make no effort to obtain doctors' permission nor do they interfere with residents who may wish to drink as long as these residents have physician permission. "Discouraged" implies that the staff directly attempt to prevent people from consuming alcohol or discourage physicians from giving their permission. "Intolerable" means that a person who drank, even with a physician's permission, would probably be asked to move.

Items 4, 5, and 7: Questions With Alternatives. These items ask about two separate possessions or behaviors. If there are different policies for the two items in a single question, credit the facility with the more liberal policy. For example, if residents are allowed to have a fish in their room but are discouraged from having a bird, mark allowed. The logic here is that the facility allows some flexibility or choice and should be credited for it.

Item 10: Locking Doors. If rooms do not have locks on doors, mark this item intolerable.

*Section III, Part III: Expectations Relating
to Level of Functional Ability; and Part IV:
Rules Related to Potential "Problem" Behaviors*

For Parts III and IV, the categories are allowed, tolerated, discouraged, and intolerable. Encouraged is not available as a category because these behaviors or lessened abilities are presumably never encouraged.

*Section III, Part V:
Resident Participation*

Item 1: Residents' Jobs in the Facility. This item applies only to people who were residents before they were hired for jobs in the facility and not people who were employees and then moved into the facility.

Item 2: Residents' Unpaid Chores. The unpaid chores or duties might include clerical or receptionist work, housework, gardening, or coordinating social functions.

Item 5a: Residents' Committees. These committees can include those for social events, entertainment, food, grievances, policy, and facility appearance.

Item 7a: Bulletin Board. You may be able to tell that the bulletin board is used by residents; if not, ask.

Section III, Part VI:
Decision Making

If there are no regulations or the administration exercises no control over specific areas of the resident's life (e.g., concerning visiting hours or participation in activities), mark Category 4 to indicate that residents basically decide by themselves. If the facility has no meal plan, mark Category 4 for Items 6 and 7.

Section IV:
Services and Activities Available

Questions on the availability and use of services are included in this section. Information on the number of residents using the services is an optional part of the POLIF. Determine whether this information will be used before completing this section of the POLIF. Include or omit these questions accordingly. To complete this part, use record sheets to tabulate the approximate numbers of residents using the available services in a typical week. These records are generally kept by the person in charge of the service. If records are not available, ask a knowledgeable staff member to estimate the number of residents who use each service in a typical week.

Section IV, Part I: Services

Item 1: Doctor's Hours. Regularly scheduled doctor's hours are scheduled hours when a physician is at the facility and available to see residents. Available hours must be at least weekly to be credited here. Do not count visits to the resident by the resident's personal physician.

Item 2: Doctor on Call. If the facility contracts with a physician who will, if called, come to the facility to see any resident, then the service is available. This service should be credited even if the resident is charged an extra fee for the service. This service is usually used only in an emergency.

Item 3: Nurse's Hours. To credit nurse's hours, they must be scheduled at least weekly. Include public health nurses who visit the facility at least once a week to see residents. If a facility has a professionally trained staff nurse who interacts directly with residents, then mark this item yes.

Item 5: Medical Clinic. Credit the facility if it has an equipped medical clinic on the grounds available for resident use.

Items 6 through 10: Therapy and Counseling Services. Count therapy and counseling services as available if the facility offers them to residents directly, either through its own staff or through consultants hired by the facility, even if residents are charged extra for the service. Do not count referrals as providing the service. Do not count such services if provided by someone not trained to deliver them or by someone whose job description does not include these duties. For example, if a bookkeeper or gardener gives religious advice to residents, do not consider this a provided service; similarly, do not consider an employee who takes residents for a walk to be providing physical therapy. Note that a member of the clergy who conducts services within the facility is not providing religious counseling; religious services are counted in Part III.

Item 12: Housekeeping Assistance. Assistance with housekeeping or cleaning can range from a weekly light housekeeping service to complete maid service.

Item 13: Preparing Meals. Credit assistance with preparing meals only when the staff help residents cook their own meals. Do not count dining room service.

Item 14: Personal Care. Personal care can range from minimal, such as standing by to assist residents as they dress or bathe, to complete personal care.

Item 15: Beauty Service. Credit this service when the facility arranges to have a barber or beautician come into the facility, even if residents must pay extra.

Item 16: Laundry Service. Count this service if the facility takes responsibility for any of the residents' laundry ranging from bed linens only to all linens and personal laundry.

Item 17: Shopping Assistance. This service ranges from having a staff member accompany residents while they shop to shopping done for individual residents.

Item 18: Transportation. Include both personal and business transportation if arranged by the facility—for example, rides to a shopping center or doctor's visit.

Section IV, Part II:
Additional Services and Procedures

Items 1, 2, and 3: Meals Served. If the meal is served Monday through Friday, check the box labeled "M-F only."

Items 1a, 2a, and 3a: Hours of Meal Service. Indicate the times during which a resident can eat a specific meal. These questions tap the choice and flexibility residents are allowed in scheduling their mealtimes. For example, if residents can pick up their lunch tray or be served lunch any time between 12:00 and 1:30, these are the hours lunch is available. If residents are brought a tray sometime between 12:00 and 1:30 but do not control when they are served during this period, however, indicate that meals are served at 12:00 and do not list a range of times. In some cases, two mealtimes may be scheduled—for example, a 5:30 dinner and a 7:00 dinner. If residents can choose which meal to attend, then list the time range as "5:30 to 7:00." If they cannot choose, record this as "5:30 or 7:00."

Item 5: Seating at Meals. If residents determine their own seating at meals, answer this question yes even if they sit in the same seat every day. If the staff determine seating at meals, either by placing name tags at seats or by directing residents to particular seats, answer this question no.

Items 7, 8, and 9: Set Times. These questions measure whether residents are free to determine their own daily schedule or whether the staff determine this schedule for residents. If bath times vary from one day to another, but the staff determine when a resident will be bathed, answer

Question 8 yes. In recording when residents are awakened or expected to go to bed, use the earliest time at which these occur.

Item 10: Curfew. This question focuses on the time in the evening when residents are expected to be in the facility of their own accord or when relatives or friends are requested to return residents to the facility.

Item 13: Visiting Hours. This question is concerned with the visiting hours residents are allowed. Answer no if the facility does not govern the time or length of stay for visitors.

Item 14: Private Offices. If you can hear what people in an office are saying when you are standing outside the closed door, mark no.

Item 15: Background Music. Mark yes if music is piped into any part of the building used by residents. Even if the music is played only some of the time or in some of the rooms, mark yes.

Section IV, Part III:
Activities That Take Place in the Facility

Ask the person responsible for organizing, coordinating, or advertising activities to give you activity schedules or calendars for the preceding months. Ascertain the central purpose or focus of the activity and classify it accordingly; do not count incidental or secondary activities such as the reality orientation that occurs during most activities. Where the nature of the activity is ambiguous, discuss it with the activity person so you can classify it in one of the categories provided in Part III. Count a given activity in only one category.

For activities in large facilities, indicate the number of people who participate in the activity at one time or another. In smaller facilities, go through the list of activities for each resident and check off those in which the resident participates. To determine the number of residents who participate, add the number of residents who attend or participate in the activity at some time. For example, if several discussion groups are held, the number participating would be the number who attend at least one. If a person attends all the discussion groups, however, count his or her attendance only once.

6 🏠

SHELTERED CARE
ENVIRONMENT SCALE

The social climate perspective assumes that every environment has a unique "personality" that gives it unity and coherence. Like people, some social environments are friendlier than others. Just as people differ in how they regulate their own behavior, settings vary in how they regulate the behavior of the people in them. Individuals form global ideas about an environment from their appraisal of specific aspects of it. For example, a judgment of friendliness might stem from whether residents greet each other in the lounge, help each other, participate in activities, and so on. These conditions establish the social climate or atmosphere of a setting.

The Sheltered Care Environment Scale (SCES) is composed of 63 yes/no items that measure the social climate of residential settings for older adults. It is one of a set of 10 scales that measure the social climate of a variety of settings including families, the workplace, and psychiatric treatment programs (Moos, 1994). The SCES assesses a facility's social environment by asking residents and staff about the usual patterns of behavior there. In contrast with other parts of the Multiphasic Environmental Assessment Procedure (MEAP), it taps participants' appraisal of their environment rather than objective information about it. The content of the SCES overlaps with the other measures but is more evaluative. For example, physical comfort is measured by questions such as "Is the furniture comfortable and homey?" and "Is it ever cold and drafty?" Resident influence is measured by such questions as "Can residents change things if they really try?" and "Do residents have any say in making the rules?" Because the SCES measures the appraised environ-

TABLE 6.1 Sheltered Care Environment Scale (SCES) Subscale Descriptions

Subscale	Description
	Relationship dimensions
Cohesion	How helpful and supportive staff members are toward residents and how involved and supportive residents are with each other
Conflict	The extent to which residents express anger and are critical of each other and of the facility
	Personal growth dimensions
Independence	How self-sufficient residents are encouraged to be and how much responsibility they exercise
Self-Disclosure	The extent to which residents openly express their feelings and personal concerns
	System maintenance and change dimensions
Organization	The extent to which residents know what to expect in their daily routines and the clarity of rules and procedures
Resident Influence	The extent to which residents can influence the facility policies and are free from restrictive regulations
Physical Comfort	The extent to which comfort, privacy, pleasant decor, and sensory satisfaction are provided by the physical environment

ment, completed questionnaires are solicited from as many respondents as possible. Individual reports are then aggregated into facility scores.

The SCES has two forms: The Real Form (Form R) measures residents' and staff members' views of the facility, and the Ideal Form (Form I) assesses preferences about residential settings.

SCES SUBSCALES

The seven SCES subscales measure three sets of dimensions (see Table 6.1). The first two subscales assess relationship dimensions. Cohesion measures how involved and supportive staff members are toward residents and how involved residents are with each other. Conflict taps the extent to which residents express anger and are critical of each other and of the facility.

The next two subscales tap personal growth or goal orientation dimensions. Independence measures how self-sufficient residents are encouraged to be and how much responsibility they exercise. Self-disclosure reflects the extent to which they openly discuss their feelings and personal concerns.

The last three subscales assess system maintenance and change dimensions. Organization measures how orderly the facility program is, whether residents know what to expect in their day-to-day routine, and the clarity of rules and procedures. Resident Influence evaluates the degree to which residents can influence policies and the extent to which residents are free from restrictive regulations. Physical Comfort taps the comfort, privacy, pleasant decor, and sensory satisfaction provided by the physical environment.

NORMATIVE SAMPLES AND
PSYCHOMETRIC CHARACTERISTICS

Normative Samples

Normative data for the SCES are available for two samples of facilities for older adults: 262 community facilities and 81 facilities serving veterans (see Normative Samples in Chapter 1). Each subscale has nine dichotomous items; raw scores are expressed as the average percentage of the nine items answered in the scored direction. Additional information about the development of the SCES is given in Lemke and Moos (1987).

The SCES itself is contained in Appendix A, hand-scoring worksheets are provided in Appendix B, and tables for converting raw percentage scores to standard scores are in Appendix C.

Community Facilities

We obtained SCES data from more than 1,900 residents and 2,000 staff in 124 nursing homes, from more than 1,200 residents and 390 staff in 56 residential care facilities, and from more than 2,900 residents and 270 staff in 65 congregate apartments. Means and standard deviations for the seven SCES subscales for the total community sample and for each of the three subsamples are reported for residents in Table 6.2 and for staff in Table 6.3. These data show that the SCES discriminates both between and within types of residential settings.

Compared with residential care facility and apartment residents, nursing home residents report higher conflict and lower organization and

TABLE 6.2 SCES Subscale Means and Standard Deviations for the Total Community Sample and the Three Subsamples (Residents)

Subscale	Total Sample (n = 241 Facilities)		Nursing Homes (n = 122 Facilities)		Residential Care (n = 54 Facilities)		Apartments (n = 65 Facilities)	
	Mean	SD	Mean	SD	Mean	SD	Mean	SD
Cohesion	63	12	62	12	65	13	65	13
Conflict	33	13	37	13	29	13	29	13
Independence	51	12	47	11	48	14	60	10
Self-Disclosure	36	9	34	9	35	11	38	7
Organization	69	11	65	10	72	11	73	11
Resident Influence	44	10	43	11	45	11	44	7
Physical Comfort	81	11	75	10	85	11	88	8

physical comfort. Similarly, compared with staff in other facilities, nursing home staff characterize these settings as higher on conflict and lower on cohesion, organization, and physical comfort. Residents and staff in the apartments score higher on resident's independence than do respondents in the other types of facilities.

Comparisons of average resident and staff perceptions show that staff see much more emphasis on conflict, self-disclosure, and resident influ-

TABLE 6.3 SCES Subscale Means and Standard Deviations for the Total Community Sample and the Three Subsamples (Staff)

Subscale	Total Sample (n = 234 Facilities)		Nursing Homes (n = 123 Facilities)		Residential Care (n = 53 Facilities)		Apartments (n = 58 Facilities)	
	Mean	SD	Mean	SD	Mean	SD	Mean	SD
Cohesion	72	12	69	11	75	14	75	13
Conflict	57	17	64	12	49	19	50	18
Independence	58	14	54	10	55	15	68	16
Self-Disclosure	61	13	63	10	60	15	58	15
Organization	66	14	61	12	73	14	72	14
Resident Influence	60	12	60	9	60	16	60	13
Physical Comfort	77	15	68	12	86	12	87	11

TABLE 6.4   SCES Subscale Means and Standard Deviations for the Total
Veterans Sample and the Two Subsamples (Residents)

Subscale	Total Sample (n = 81 Facilities)		Nursing Care Units (n = 57 Facilities)		Domiciliaries (n = 24 Facilities)	
	Mean	SD	Mean	SD	Mean	SD
Cohesion	55	10	56	10	54	9
Conflict	47	13	44	12	54	14
Independence	46	10	45	10	48	7
Self-Disclosure	37	9	34	8	43	9
Organization	60	11	59	11	60	11
Resident Influence	40	9	40	9	38	10
Physical Comfort	70	13	70	14	69	13

ence and somewhat more cohesion and independence than do residents.
Average staff and resident perceptions are relatively similar for organization and physical comfort. Other researchers have found a similar
pattern of differences between the perceptions of residents and staff in
nursing homes (e.g., Stein, Linn, & Stein, 1987).

Veterans Facilities

We obtained SCES data from 786 residents and 1,077 staff in 57
veterans nursing care units and from 759 residents and 262 staff in 24
domiciliaries. The SCES means and standard deviations for the sample
of 81 veterans facilities and for each of the two subsamples are given in
Table 6.4 for residents and in Table 6.5 for staff.

Comparisons of the subsamples of veterans facilities indicate that
domiciliary residents report higher conflict and self-disclosure than do
residents in the veterans nursing care units. In other respects, the social
climates are quite similar. The differences in staff perceptions between
the two types of veterans facilities are generally larger than those shown
for residents. Compared with staff in veterans nursing care units, staff in
the domiciliaries report higher cohesion, independence, organization,
and physical comfort and lower conflict and resident influence.

Paralleling the pattern found in community facilities, staff in veterans
facilities report more conflict, self-disclosure, and resident influence than

TABLE 6.5   SCES Subscale Means and Standard Deviations for the Total
Veterans Sample and the Two Subsamples (Staff)

Subscale	Total Sample (n = 80 Facilities)		Nursing Care Units (n = 57 Facilities)		Domiciliaries (n = 23 Facilities)	
	Mean	SD	Mean	SD	Mean	SD
Cohesion	60	11	58	11	65	12
Conflict	71	11	74	8	66	15
Independence	46	13	42	11	56	12
Self-Disclosure	56	11	56	9	54	13
Organization	54	13	51	13	61	12
Resident Influence	58	12	61	9	50	14
Physical Comfort	55	16	51	15	64	15

do residents. Compared with residents, domiciliary staff also report somewhat higher levels of cohesion and independence; residents and staff in nursing home units tend to agree with one another on the overall levels of these characteristics. Although the overall levels of organization and physical comfort are similar for residents and staff in the community sample, staff in the nursing home units are more critical than are the residents of these aspects of the setting.

Comparing veterans and community nursing facilities, we find substantial differences in their social climates. In general, residents and staff in the veterans nursing care units report more conflict, poorer organization, and less cohesion and physical comfort than do residents and staff in community nursing homes. In addition, staff in the veterans nursing care units report less independence than do staff in community nursing homes. Residents and staff in the domiciliaries tend to report more conflict and less cohesion, organization, resident influence, and physical comfort than do the residential care residents and staff.

Differences Among Facilities

In addition to the differences between types of facilities, there are substantial differences among facilities of one type. One-way analysis of variance for each subsample indicates that all seven subscales discriminate significantly ($p < .05$) between facilities for residents in nursing

TABLE 6.6 SCES Subscale Internal Consistency, Split-Half Reliability, and Test-Retest Reliability

Subscale	Internal Consistency[a]		Split-Sample Reliability[b]	
	Residents	Staff	Residents	Staff
Cohesion	.65	.73	.86	.67
Conflict	.76	.76	.80	.78
Independence	.60	.69	.80	.65
Self-Disclosure	.59	.68	.66	.59
Organization	.66	.74	.82	.69
Resident Influence	.44	.56	.69	.67
Physical Comfort	.76	.79	.90	.83

a. $n = 1,041$ residents and $n = 792$ staff.
b. $n = 52$ facilities for residents and $n = 66$ facilities for staff.

homes, residential care facilities, and apartments. Similar results were obtained for staff in the nursing homes and apartments. For staff in residential care facilities, all subscales except organization showed significantly more variation between facilities than within them.

Subscale Internal Consistencies and Intercorrelations

Table 6.6 shows the subscale internal consistencies (Cronbach's alpha) for a representative group of residents and staff. The sample was selected by using data from up to eight residents and eight staff in each facility assessed in phase two of the project. Six of the seven SCES subscales have acceptable to high internal consistency. Internal consistency is only moderate for the Resident Influence subscale. Examination of the pattern of item intercorrelations suggests that two issues are being tapped by this dimension. One is whether the facility is open to change in response to resident input ("Do residents have any say in making the rules?"), and the other is how strict the staff are in enforcing regulations ("Would a resident ever be asked to leave if he or she broke a rule?"). Although both issues concern residents' power in the facility, in practice they appear to be only loosely related.

Split-sample reliabilities were computed for 52 facilities in which 20 or more residents completed questionnaires. For staff, they were based on results from 66 facilities in which 10 or more questionnaires were

TABLE 6.7 Partial Correlations Among SCES Subscales, With Level of Care Controlled[a]

Subscale	Cohesion	Conflict	Independence	Self-Disclosure	Organization	Resident Influence	Physical Comfort
Cohesion	(.38)	−.37	.44	−.12	.52	.21	.48
Conflict	−.28	(.43)	−.13	.48	−.51	.04	−.47
Independence	.50	−.21	(.38)	.04	.25	.22	.25
Self-Disclosure	.13	.35	.10	(.22)	−.28	.12	−.26
Organization	.59	−.45	.35	−.03	(.48)	.08	.58
Resident Influence	.11	.07	.17	.18	.05	(.27)	.10
Physical Comfort	.52	−.46	.33	−.04	.57	.01	(.36)

a. Correlations above the diagonal (the diagonal is the numbers in parentheses) are for a representative set of residents ($n = 1,085$); those below the diagonal are for a representative sample of staff ($n = 826$). Correlations along the diagonal are between residents and staff for the 227 community facilities in which both groups completed the SCES.

available. Split-sample reliabilities were calculated by computing the correlation between the facility score obtained from half the respondents and that obtained from the remainder (odd vs. even cases). These reliability coefficients are reported in Table 6.6; they are moderate to high, indicating that SCES results are relatively independent of the particular sample of individuals responding.

The intercorrelations among the seven subscales (partial correlations of individual scores with the type of facility controlled) are shown in Table 6.7. The subscale intercorrelations for residents, which are shown above the diagonal, are moderate (three of the correlations are above .50); those for staff, which are shown below the diagonal, are roughly similar (four of the intercorrelations are above .50). In general, Cohesion, Independence, Organization, and Physical Comfort are positively interrelated, whereas Conflict shows negative correlations with these dimensions. The average subscale correlations ($r = .28$ for residents and .26 for staff) are moderate, indicating that the SCES subscales tap somewhat separate but interrelated aspects of the social climate of a facility.

Correlations between residents and staff for the subscale means in the 227 community facilities that have questionnaires from both groups indicate that these two groups are in moderate agreement concerning the social climate of their facility (see the diagonal of Table 6.7). Because these two groups may have quite different perspectives, and the extent of resident-staff agreement varies from one facility to another, it is useful to obtain the views of both groups.

Test-Retest Reliability and Profile Stability

We obtained subscale and profile stability data by readministering the SCES in 12 facilities after an interval of 9 to 12 months. The stability was moderate to high for five of the seven subscales, but Self-Disclosure and Resident Influence varied considerably over a year's time.

We also computed the profile stability for each of these 12 facilities, and the resulting correlations ranged from .09 to .96 for residents (mean $r = .57$) and from .21 to .85 for staff (mean $r = .60$). Given the split-sample reliabilities, the low profile stabilities in some facilities appear to reflect real changes in people's perceptions of their environment rather than simply differences in who responds to the questionnaire (e.g., see the discussion of Woodside Nursing Home, which was one of the facilities with a low profile stability, on pp. 129-130).

THE IDEAL FORM

We developed the Ideal Form of the SCES (SCES Form I) to measure the value orientations of residents and staff. The SCES Form I is composed of SCES items and instructions reworded to describe an ideal residential facility. The SCES Form I has 63 items, each of which is parallel to an item in Form R. The SCES Form I helps residents and staff describe the type of residential facility they would like. Other respondents, such as family members or older people residing in their own homes, can complete the SCES Form I.

The SCES Form I has many applications. It can facilitate comparison of preferences of different groups, for example, by revealing similarities and differences between staff and resident goals or between preferences of current and prospective residents. When used in conjunction with Form R, Form I helps to measure person-environment congruence. Such comparisons can identify areas in which residents and staff feel that change should occur. (For more information about potential applications, see Brennan, Moos, & Lemke, 1988, 1989; Moos & Lemke, 1984; Moos, Lemke, & Clayton, 1983; Moos, Lemke, & David, 1987.)

TABLE 6.8 SCES Form I Subscale Means and Standard Deviations for
             Residents and Staff

Subscale	Total Sample of Residents $(n = 90)$[a]		Total Sample of Staff $(n = 55)$[b]	
	Mean	SD	Mean	SD
Cohesion	76	16	78	18
Conflict	16	17	46	27
Independence	77	16	71	18
Self-Disclosure	31	21	64	22
Organization	82	17	74	21
Resident Influence	49	16	61	21
Physical Comfort	95	10	82	19

a. Residents were sampled from residential care facilities and apartments.
b. Staff were sampled from residential care facilities and nursing homes.

The items and instructions for the SCES Form I appear in Appendix D; Form I can be used with the same answer sheet, scoring template, and scoring instructions as those used for Form R.

Normative Samples

We obtained data on the SCES Form I from 90 residents (44 in residential care facilities and 46 in apartments) and 55 staff members (29 in nursing homes and 26 in residential care facilities). Given the small size of these samples, we distinguish between residents and staff but not by facility type (see Table 6.8). As expected, residents and staff desire high levels of cohesion, independence, and physical comfort. Organization receives high ratings as well, with residents giving it a stronger endorsement than do staff. Also as we expected, both residents and staff describe the ideal residential facility as low on conflict, but residents prefer much less than do the staff. In addition, staff express a much higher preference for self-disclosure and resident influence than do residents.

These differences must be interpreted with caution due to the small number of cases and the fact that residents were sampled from residential care facilities and apartments, whereas staff were sampled from residential care facilities and nursing homes.

USING THE SCES TO
DESCRIBE GROUP RESIDENCES

The SCES has been widely used in characterizing facilities and evaluating programs. Here, we present SCES profile interpretations and illustrate the comparison of actual and preferred social climates. The SCES provides reliable information about a facility and can help residents and staff become involved in program planning and change. Program evaluators can obtain additional information about a facility by giving the SCES to outside observers or family members and comparing their views with those of residents and staff (Jones & Batterson, 1982).

When Form R and Form I are both used, they can alert administrators to discrepancies between a facility's social climate and resident or staff preferences. When used with the other MEAP instruments, the SCES can help characterize the quality of a residential setting. Chapters 1 and 8 detail these and other MEAP applications.

Profile Interpretation

To illustrate the interpretation of facility profiles, we present profiles of the three facilities introduced in Chapter 3. Results are shown as standard scores with a mean of 50 and a standard deviation of 10. (For additional examples of SCES profiles, see Moos & Lemke, 1983, 1994; Moos et al., 1983.)

City Haven Nursing Home

City Haven, an urban nursing home, had undergone a change in ownership almost a year prior to the assessment. Although residents are fairly typical of nursing home residents in their backgrounds and current functioning, they are relatively inactive. On the SCES, residents report a moderate level of interpersonal engagement. As shown in Figure 6.1, cohesion is about average and conflict is reported to be somewhat high. Staff report an even higher level of conflict, but they also report a high level of positive engagement.

Residents feel that they exercise above-average independence and are very open about their feelings and personal problems (high independence and self-disclosure). Here again, staff are in moderate agreement; they, too, report high independence but see self-disclosure as only slightly above average, perhaps because the activities that focus on reminiscence

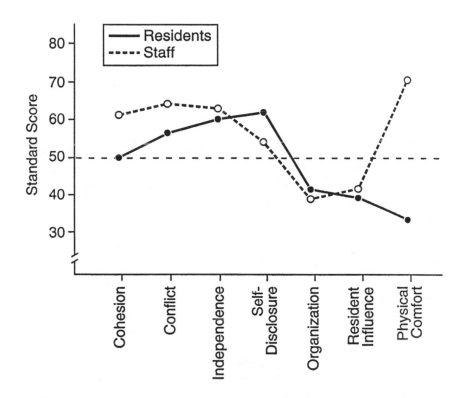

Figure 6.1. Social Climate Profile for City Haven Nursing Home

and sharing of feelings are brought into the facility by a community agency.

Residents and staff report that City Haven is disorganized and that residents have little influence on policies and are restricted by the rules. As noted, City Haven was in the process of establishing new routines in response to the ownership change and subsequent turnover in staff. In addition, the lack of clarity in communicating expectations, shown in the Policy and Program Information Form (POLIF) profile, may have contributed to the perception of poor organization. The POLIF profile also shows below-average levels of policy choice, resident control, and privacy, which may help account for the low score on the Resident Influence subscale.

Finally, City Haven residents were critical of the facility's comfort. In contrast, staff members saw City Haven as a very pleasant environment. The difference in their views may reflect the ample provision of staff facilities and relatively limited physical resources for residents.

El Dorado Residential Care Facility

As part of a nonprofit, life-care facility, El Dorado serves a group of residents who are mostly older women from lower socioeconomic backgrounds. The older building in which it is housed is rich in resources and provides access to the community, numerous amenities and recreational features, features to ensure safety, and ample space allowances and privacy. The policies set high expectations for resident functioning, and the services emphasize health care rather than assistance with daily living tasks.

Residents and staff of El Dorado have a relatively high level of consensus regarding the social climate of their facility (Figure 6.2). Both groups see relationships as quite cohesive and conflict as about average.

Staff and residents have somewhat different views of the emphasis on independence. Residents report an above-average level of independence, whereas staff report it to be about average. Compared with staff, residents are more likely to report that they are taught new skills and less likely to say that they depend on staff to set up activities for them. Both groups say that self-disclosure is about average.

Residents think the facility is very well run and efficient. From the point of view of staff, organization is about average. Although policies provide only average levels of choice and control, staff and residents agree that residents have a high level of influence. Staff, however, are more likely than residents to say that the rules are not strictly enforced. Consistent with the many physical resources available, both groups rate the facility as comfortable and pleasant.

Marlborough Arms Apartments

Marlborough Arms is a small, privately operated apartment complex. Although recently constructed, it offers the physical resources found in most such facilities. The policies permit a moderate level of disability,

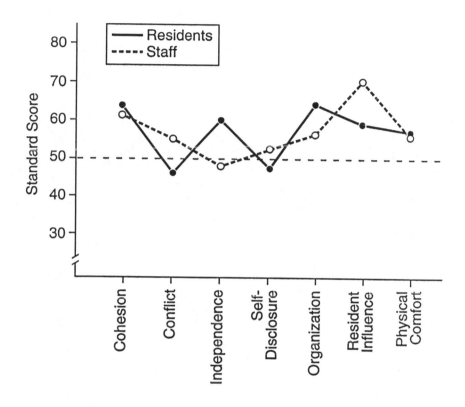

Figure 6.2. Social Climate Profile for El Dorado Residential Care Facility

and the resident population is consequently somewhat more impaired than average. The facility offers more health services and assistance in daily activities than are typical. Provisions for choice and privacy are about average, but opportunities for a formal voice in facility decision making are limited.

Residents and staff of Marlborough Arms agree in some respects in their view of the facility's social climate but have marked differences in

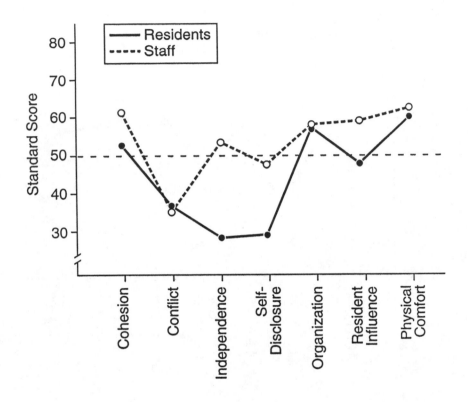

Figure 6.3. Social Climate Profile for Marlborough Arms Apartments

others (Figure 6.3). Staff rate cohesion above average and somewhat higher than residents do. Both groups see a very low level of conflict.

Their views of program emphasis are markedly different. Residents report that the emphasis on independence and self-disclosure is very low, whereas staff see it as about average. Unlike residents, staff report that residents sometimes take charge of activities and are taught how to deal with practical problems. Similarly, staff members say that personal problems are openly talked about and that residents talk about illness and death, but few residents agree.

Both groups see organization as slightly above average and physical comfort as above average, but they disagree on the level of resident influence. Staff report an above-average level of resident influence and say that residents have a voice in making the rules. Residents disagree and report an average level of influence.

Comparing Actual and Preferred Social Climates

Information about preferences is useful in planning interventions designed to change a facility. When used together, Forms R and I of the SCES can help to clarify the values of residents and staff and point to discrepancies between the actual environment and people's ideals.

To illustrate, we present SCES results from Peachtree Manor, a federally assisted apartment facility that had been open for about 1 year. Located in a rural area, it is somewhat isolated from community resources. The 125 residents are in most respects typical of apartment facility residents: Their average age is 75, 80% are women, and 60% are widowed. Fewer than 20% have any education beyond high school, however, and nearly all had been homemakers or had held blue-collar or clerical jobs. The residents are relatively homogeneous in background and, despite the distance, frequently go into the community for activities.

The SCES Form R results, shown in Figure 6.4, indicate that residents see relationships as friendly and relatively free of conflict. They report average emphasis on resident independence but somewhat below-average emphasis on self-disclosure. They see the facility as comfortable and orderly but report that they have little control over policies or input in decisions.

The SCES Form I profile for these residents, also shown in Figure 6.4, is like their actual environment in most respects. Residents are mostly satisfied with the friendliness of relationships, the facility's organization, and its physical environment. They express, however, a desire for less conflict, less emphasis on self-disclosure, and more independence and resident influence.

In a private long-term care facility, Waters (1980a) administered the Real and Ideal Forms of the SCES to nursing and social services staff. The social services staff and the residents perceived high cohesion and independence, but the nursing staff perceived just average emphasis on all of the dimensions. Real-Ideal discrepancy scores indicated that the

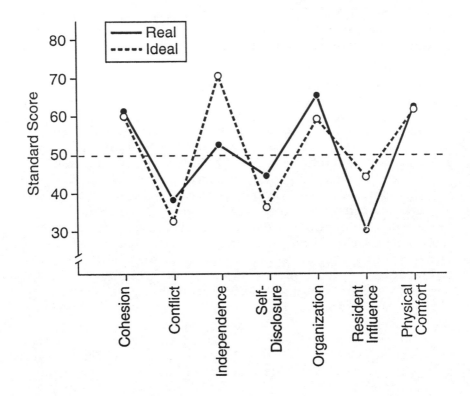

Figure 6.4. Social Climate for Peachtree Manor Apartments and Preferences of Its Residents

staff wanted more emphasis on cohesion, independence, organization, and physical comfort and less on conflict (see also Waters, 1980b).

Monitoring Changes in Social Climate

Administrators and staff can use the SCES to monitor a facility over time, to suggest program modifications, and to evaluate the results of change efforts. For example, assessment of a residential facility's social climate can alert an evaluator that the program fails to accomplish desired objectives, as when the administrator reports the existence of a residents' council and high resident participation in decision making but residents report that they have little influence on facility policies. Chapters 1 and 8 provide more specific information about these applications.

The SCES is sensitive to naturally occurring changes such as those that may accompany a change in facility management. For example, residents and staff in Woodside Nursing Home completed the SCES on one occasion and then again 3 and 4 years later. Initially, this home was owned by a small corporation and had had the same administrator for more than 10 years. Just prior to the second assessment, the home was sold to a large, out-of-state corporation, and a new administrator took over. The final assessment was made in the following year when the administrator had changed again and there were rumors of an impending sale.

Figure 6.5 shows the staff profiles at the initial assessment and at the final assessment 4 years later. Initially, staff viewed this nursing home as slightly above average on cohesion, independence, and organization and average on the remaining dimensions (see Figure 6.5). Three years later, immediately after the sale, staff scored about average on all dimensions except resident influence, which was above average. One year after that, the facility scored very low on all dimensions except conflict.

Discussions with staff at the final assessment revealed very low morale; the head nurse reported increased absenteeism and tardiness, and long-time aides said they were ready to quit. Complaints centered on the change in administrative philosophy from patient to profit centered, with accompanying shortages of supplies, overwork, and lack of responsiveness to staff complaints. Staff members stated that they were striving to maintain the same quality of care, but they were highly critical of the new administrator and owners. Resident perceptions were relatively stable over this period, although self-disclosure and resident influence declined substantially. Thus, staff were relatively successful in buffering residents from the changes they had experienced.

ADMINISTRATION OF THE SCES

Because many people must cooperate in the completion of the SCES, you will need to take particular care in presenting it, in setting up procedures for its administration, and in obtaining resident and staff

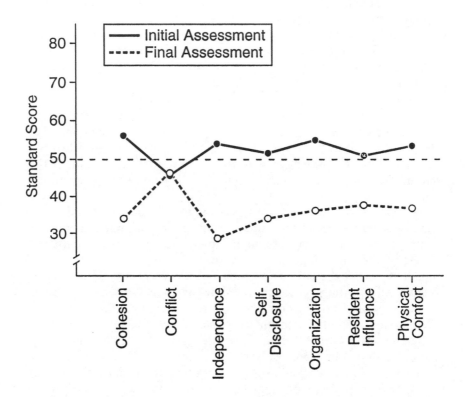

Figure 6.5. Staff Social Climate for Longitudinal Assessment of Woodside Nursing Home

cooperation. It may help if you point out that the SCES provides unique information about how staff and residents feel about the facility. Decide in advance whether you will provide feedback to each facility on the SCES results. If you plan to do so, emphasize this benefit of participation. Chapter 2 provides suggestions for presenting the MEAP to facility administrators and staff, setting policies about confidentiality and the use of the MEAP results, and encouraging cooperation in the data collection process.

Practically achievable response rates from residents vary considerably among facilities. Usually, over 60% of residents in group homes, domiciliaries, and apartment buildings can complete the SCES. In facilities in which residents' functional abilities are low or literacy is a problem, however, the return rate can be as low as 20% to 40%. In the majority of nursing homes, a 20% response rate can be achieved, although rates may vary from 10% to 40%. Achieving high response rates from staff is generally a question of adequately motivating them.

Try to obtain at least 10 completed questionnaires from residents and at least 5 from staff members. A completed questionnaire is one on which no more than 10 questions are unanswered. Split-sample reliabilities with these minimum numbers of respondents are moderately high; that is, SCES results obtained with such sample sizes are relatively independent of the specific individuals responding.

If you plan to score the SCES by hand, use the answer sheet in Appendix A. In administrations to groups of staff, you can read the SCES questions aloud while staff record their responses on the answer sheets; you should monitor the staff's use of the answer sheet to ensure accuracy. You can also use the answer sheet to record responses when administering the SCES in interview format to impaired residents. If scoring will be done by computer, respondents can mark their answers directly on the questionnaire.

See Chapter 2 for suggestions regarding specific procedures for administering the SCES to residents and staff.

General Problems in Administering the SCES

The following questions or problems may arise during administration:

Respondents may say they cannot answer "yes" or "no" to a statement because it is "sometimes true and sometimes false." Tell them to answer in terms of what generally is the case: If it is *mostly* true, circle yes; if it is *mostly* false, circle no.

Respondents may say that the question is inappropriate for their facility. In such cases, the statement should generally be marked no. For example, in response to the question, "Would a resident ever be asked to leave if he or she broke a rule?," apartment residents may say that there are no rules. At other times, this response indicates that the statement is awkward or embarrassing for the person to answer. Point out that for some facilities the question can be answered yes and for others it can be answered no; try to persuade the respondent to answer the question.

The respondent may ask what a statement means. Try to explain as clearly as you can while staying close to the wording and tone of the original statement.

You may need to define the terms "resident" and "staff," particularly in medical facilities. Explain that resident means all the people who live in a facility and staff designates all the people who work there.

Be prepared to explain which items on the cover sheet should be answered and why. The questionnaire can be answered anonymously, but other information about the respondent (such as age, length of residence, and staff position) may be important for specific purposes such as longitudinal follow-up or a study of the relationship between staff role and environmental perceptions. Respondents may also wish to know who will see the completed questionnaire, how results will be compiled, and whether or not they will be shared with staff or residents (see Chapter 2 for a discussion of these issues).

7 🏠

THE RATING SCALE

The Rating Scale is composed of 24 items that tap observers' impressions of the physical environment and of resident and staff functioning in a residential facility. The content of the Rating Scale overlaps with the Resident and Staff Information Form (RESIF) and Physical and Architectural Features Checklist (PAF) but is intended to tap more subjective aspects of the setting such as its attractiveness, the involvement of residents, and the quality of staff interactions with residents.

SUBSCALES OF THE RATING SCALE

The four Rating Scale subscales are presented in Table 7.1. Physical Attractiveness is composed of ratings of the facility grounds and buildings as well as of the noise level, odors, illumination, cleanliness, and condition of the facility. Environmental Diversity reflects the extent to which the physical environment provides stimulation and variety; this subscale includes ratings of the window areas, the views from the windows, the variation and personalization of residents' rooms, and the distinctiveness of living spaces.

The Resident Functioning subscale summarizes evaluations of residents' appearance, activity level, and interaction. The Staff Functioning subscale reflects the quality of interaction between staff and residents, the organization of the facility, and the amount of conflict among staff members. All items on the Rating Scale are rated and scored on 4-point scales.

TABLE 7.1 Rating Scale Subscale Descriptions

Subscale	Description
	Physical environment
Physical Attractiveness	The cleanliness, condition, and esthetic appeal of the facility
Environmental Diversity	The variety and stimulation provided by the physical environment
	Residents and staff
Resident Functioning	The appearance, activity level, and interactions of residents
Staff Functioning	The quality of interaction between staff and residents, the organization of the facility, and the relationships among the staff

NORMATIVE SAMPLES AND PSYCHOMETRIC CHARACTERISTICS

Normative Samples

Normative data for the Rating Scale were obtained from two samples of facilities for older adults: 262 community facilities and 81 facilities serving veterans (see Normative Samples in Chapter 1).

The raw scores represent the percentage of the total possible points the observers have credited to the facility. For example, the Physical Attractiveness subscale is composed of nine items. A facility can potentially obtain 3 points on each item for a total of 27 points. Table 7.2 shows that, on average, facilities obtained 68% of the possible points on Physical Attractiveness.

The Rating Scale is contained in Appendix A, hand-scoring worksheets are in Appendix B, and directions for converting raw percentage scores to standard scores are in Appendix C.

Community Facilities

Means and standard deviations for the four Rating Scale subscales for the total community sample and for each of the three subsamples are reported in Table 7.2. The sample of community facilities varied on all four Rating Scale subscales as shown by the standard deviations in Table 7.2.

TABLE 7.2 Rating Scale Subscale Means and Standard Deviations for the
Total Community Sample and Three Subsamples

Subscale	Total Sample (n = 262 Facilities)		Nursing Homes (n = 135 Facilities)		Residential Care (n = 60 Facilities)		Apartments (n = 67 Facilities)	
	Mean	SD	Mean	SD	Mean	SD	Mean	SD
Physical Attractiveness	68	14	66	12	69	16	71	16
Environmental Diversity	60	18	52	17	61	17	74	11
Resident Functioning	68	21	59	18	69	21	85	15
Staff Functioning	68	18	73	17	66	17	59	16

The three subsamples are rated about the same on Physical Attractiveness. As expected, nursing homes scored lowest on Environmental Diversity, followed by residential care facilities and then apartments. On average, Resident Functioning is lowest in the nursing homes, intermediate in the residential care facilities, and highest in the apartments. In contrast, because of their staffing levels and the amount of resident-staff contact, Staff Functioning is highest in the nursing homes, intermediate in the residential care facilities, and lowest in the apartments.

Veterans Facilities

The means and standard deviations of the four Rating Scale subscales for the veterans facilities and for the two subsamples are shown in Table 7.3. On average, the nursing care units are somewhat lower than the domiciliaries on Physical Attractiveness. As expected, the domiciliaries are higher on Resident Functioning. Ratings on Environmental Diversity and Staff Functioning differ little between nursing care units and domiciliaries.

Comparison of the veterans facilities with the corresponding community facilities indicates that the veterans facilities are lower on Environmental Diversity. In addition, the veterans nursing care units are lower than community nursing homes on Resident Functioning, and the domiciliaries are higher than the community residential care facilities on Physical Attractiveness.

TABLE 7.3 Rating Scale Subscale Means and Standard Deviations for the
Total Veterans Sample and Two Subsamples

Subscale	Total Sample (n = 81 Facilities)		Nursing Care Units (n = 57 Facilities)		Domiciliaries (n = 24 Facilities)	
	Mean	SD	Mean	SD	Mean	SD
Physical Attractiveness	72	11	69	10	77	11
Environmental Diversity	45	17	44	13	49	24
Resident Functioning	57	21	53	19	67	23
Staff Functioning	73	15	74	14	68	16

Subscale Internal Consistencies and Intercorrelations

Table 7.4 shows the number of items on each of the Rating Scale
subscales and provides estimates of internal consistency (Cronbach's
alpha). The alphas were calculated on a subsample of more than 150
community facilities. The internal consistencies are moderate to high,
especially because three of the Rating Scale subscales contain only five
items each.

The intercorrelations among the four subscales (partial correlations
controlling for level of care) for the community sample are shown above
the diagonal in Table 7.5, and intercorrelations for veterans facilities are
shown below the diagonal. For both samples, intercorrelations are moderately high, suggesting that raters tend to view these aspects of facilities

TABLE 7.4 Rating Scale Subscale Internal Consistency and Test-Retest
Reliability

Subscale	Number of Items	Internal Consistency	Test-Retest Reliability (n = 12 Facilities)
Physical Attractiveness	9	.82	.66
Environmental Diversity	5	.73	.62
Resident Functioning	5	.82	.94
Staff Functioning	5	.67	.34

TABLE 7.5 Partial Correlations Among Rating Scale Subscales, With Level of
Care Controlled[a]

Subscale	Physical Attractiveness	Environmental Diversity	Resident Functioning	Staff Functioning
Physical Attractiveness	—	.52	.62	.45
Environmental Diversity	.57	—	.51	.33
Resident Functioning	.58	.63	—	.48
Staff Functioning	.56	.41	.48	—

a. Correlations above the diagonal are for the community sample; correlations below the diagonal are for the veterans sample.

as interrelated. Because the other Multiphasic Environmental Assessment Procedure (MEAP) subscales tend to be more independent of one another, these results suggest that observers are influenced in their individual ratings by their global impression of a facility.

Interobserver Reliability, Test-Retest Reliability, and Profile Stability

To obtain information on interobserver reliability, we had two trained project observers, two staff members, and two older community residents complete the Rating Scale in 15 facilities. The results indicate that trained observers can make reliable ratings (r varied from .71 to .84 for the four dimensions). Although facility staff and community observers agree closely with project observers on the first three Rating Scale subscales (r varied from .61 to .90), there is poor agreement on Staff Functioning. We therefore caution users against giving too much weight to ratings of Staff Functioning made by facility staff or community observers. Reliability is improved for all subscales by averaging the ratings of two independent observers.

Subscale and profile stability data were obtained by readministering the Rating Scale in 12 California facilities after an interval of 9 to 12 months. The results, shown in Table 7.4, indicate that, with the exception of Staff Functioning, the Rating Scale scores are relatively stable over time. The low test-retest correlation for Staff Functioning occurs despite high agreement between independent project observers making concurrent ratings, suggesting that staff functioning may actually be more variable than the other attributes measured by the Rating Scale.

Validity

In Chapter 1, we described how we tried to build content and face validity into the MEAP indices by formulating definitions of specific constructs, such as physical attractiveness and environmental diversity, preparing items to fit the construct definitions, and selecting items that were conceptually related to a subscale. We also examined the associations between the Rating Scale subscales and the physical features, resident and staff characteristics, and social climate in the normative sample of community facilities.

Ratings of the Physical Environment

A facility's objective physical features should be related to perceptions of its physical attractiveness and comfort. To focus on this issue, we examined the correlations between various measures of the physical environment in the community sample. Even after controlling for level of care, observers rated facilities with more physical amenities, social-recreational aids, staff facilities, and space (PAF subscales) as higher on Physical Attractiveness and Environmental Diversity. Facilities with more prosthetic and orientational aids and more safety features are rated as more attractive by observers. Thus, observers tend to rate facilities with richer physical resources as more attractive and diverse. The findings also show that the provision of supportive features need not be accompanied by a reduction in perceptions of attractiveness.

In addition, facilities that observers rated more attractive and varied are viewed as more comfortable by residents and staff (Sheltered Care Environment Scale [SCES] Physical Comfort subscale). Observers' ratings are more closely related to residents' than to staff members' perceptions of the social climate. These findings provide further evidence for the construct validity of the Rating Scale.

Ratings of Resident and Staff Functioning

We also examined the correlations between various measures of resident and staff functioning included in the MEAP. After controlling for level of care, observers' ratings of resident and staff functioning in a facility are predictably related to objectively measured staff and resident characteristics, as well as to the facility social climate.

Specifically, rated resident functioning is higher in facilities in which residents are more independent in daily activities and more involved in self-initiated activities and activities in the community. Resident functioning also is higher in facilities in which residents and staff report warmer interpersonal relations, better organization, and higher resident independence and influence. On the other hand, rated resident functioning is not related to the level of interpersonal conflict reported nor to residents' level of involvement in formal, facility-organized activities.

Ratings of staff functioning are higher in facilities in which staff resources (diversity and experience) are higher and in which staff turnover is lower. Facilities with a higher staff ratio, more women staff members, and more staff over age 50 receive slightly higher ratings of staff functioning. Staff functioning is also higher in facilities in which residents and staff report warmer relationships and better organization and in which residents see themselves as having more independence and influence. As with the physical environment, observers' ratings are more strongly related to residents' perceptions of the social climate than to staff members' perceptions.

USING THE RATING SCALE TO DESCRIBE GROUP RESIDENCES

The Rating Scale helps to describe facilities, to monitor program changes over time, and to promote program improvement. When the Rating Scale is used with other MEAP instruments, it can help characterize the quality of a residential setting. Chapters 1 and 8 describe in detail the applications of the MEAP.

Profile Interpretation

To illustrate the interpretation of facility profiles, we present Rating Scale profiles of the three community facilities introduced in Chapter 3. Results are shown as standard scores (based on the appropriate normative sample) with a mean of 50 and a standard deviation of 10.

City Haven Nursing Home

Figure 7.1 shows the Rating Scale profile for City Haven Nursing Home, an urban nursing home that had transferred ownership about 1 year before. The facility was constructed in the mid-1960s and suffers some limitations in amenities and space for residents that may reflect its

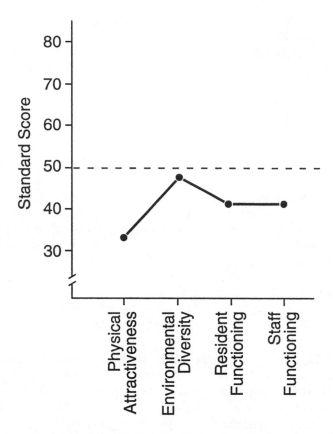

Figure 7.1. Rating Scale Profile for City Haven Nursing Home

age and urban location. As noted previously, City Haven residents are generally typical of nursing home residents in our sample in their backgrounds and current functioning, except that they are less likely to engage in informal activities.

Consistent with the PAF results and with resident perceptions of physical comfort (Figures 4.1 and 6.1), outside observers rated City Haven low on cleanliness and aesthetic appeal (low physical attractiveness). They rated it about average for a nursing home, however, in the variety and personalization provided by the building. Observers noted problems in both resident and staff functioning that may reflect residents' low activity involvement, the low staffing level and staff resources, as well as the poor organization noted by both residents and staff on the SCES.

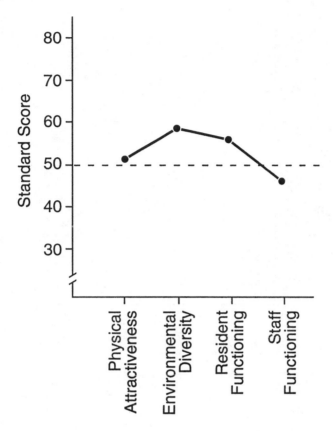

Figure 7.2. Rating Scale Profile for El Dorado Residential Care Facility

El Dorado Residential Care Facility

Figure 7.2 shows the Rating Scale profile for El Dorado Residential Care Facility, a suburban facility owned by a nonprofit group. El Dorado is seen as providing a reasonably attractive and diverse physical setting (average physical attractiveness and above-average environmental diversity). These ratings are consistent with the richness revealed by the PAF profile for this facility (Figure 4.2). The residents in this facility are rated as about average on their functioning; this is consistent with El Dorado's RESIF profile, which shows the residents to have above-average functional ability and slightly below-average activity level in the facility (Figure 3.2). Staff functioning is also typical for this type of facility.

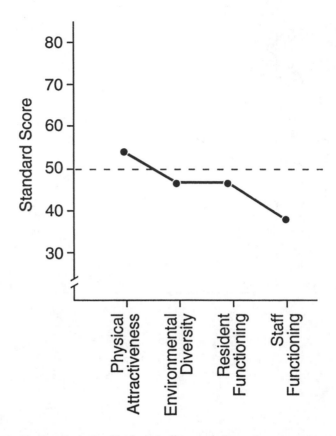

Figure 7.3. Rating Scale Profile for Marlborough Arms Apartments

Marlborough Arms Apartments

Figure 7.3 shows the Rating Scale profile for Marlborough Arms Apartments, a recently constructed, proprietary facility. The profile indicates that Marlborough Arms is about average in terms of attractiveness and diversity compared with apartment facilities. These scores are consistent with the PAF profile, which shows that this facility is about average in physical resources in most areas (Figure 4.3).

According to the Rating Scale, resident functioning at Marlborough Arms is about average and staff functioning is well below average. These findings are consistent with the RESIF profile, which shows that residents are about average in their activity involvement despite functional abilities that are well below average. The RESIF also indicates that staff are somewhat less diverse and experienced than is typical of staff in other apartment facilities (Figure 3.3).

Monitoring and Improving Programs

The Rating Scale can be used to monitor a facility over time and to evaluate the results of independently initiated program modifications. The Rating Scale is also useful in planning and evaluating interventions designed to change a facility. The Rating Scale can help administrators and staff understand important aspects of their facility, clarify how these aspects affect facility goals, and suggest ways to improve the facility (see Chapters 1 and 8).

Porter and Watson (1985) used the Rating Scale to assess 24 inpatient units at the University of Missouri-Columbia Hospital on five occasions over a 2-year period. When one unit and its grounds were renovated, the effects were reflected in increased physical attractiveness scores. Environmental diversity was especially low in the intensive care units, but one unit improved over an 18-month period as patients personalized their rooms by displaying pictures and cards on the bulletin boards and bedside tables.

Outside raters can provide a different perspective on a facility. In conjunction with an evaluation of nine residential facilities associated with a nonprofit corporation, Billingsley and Batterson (1986) asked community volunteers to use the Rating Scale to record their impressions of the facilities. The authors note that this activity provided a useful outside perspective and can help to strengthen community involvement in residential facilities. Family members can also complete the Rating Scale on the basis of their impressions of a facility, and the results can be compared with staff members' or residents' ratings.

ADMINISTRATION OF THE RATING SCALE

General Directions for the Rating Scale

Appendix A contains the Rating Scale. Most Rating Scale items can be completed while gathering information for the PAF. The remaining ratings can be made in a few minutes after completing all other data collection.

Chapter 2 provides suggestions for presenting the MEAP to facility administrators and staff, setting policies about confidentiality and the use of results, and encouraging cooperation in the data collection process.

Who Can Complete the Rating Scale

A trained observer can complete the Rating Scale using direct observation. For training, a new observer should complete practice assessments in at least three facilities, review the results with experienced observers, and discuss and resolve discrepancies. In addition, facility staff and community residents are able to complete the Rating Scale using the directions that follow. As previously noted, their ratings have good reliability except on the Staff Functioning subscale on which agreement is poor both among themselves and with trained observers. Accuracy improves if results from two observers are averaged or if the observers resolve discrepancies by mutual agreement.

Making Observations

To complete the Rating Scale, observe the facility while you take the initial tour, collect questionnaires from residents, and complete the other portions of the MEAP. Always be alert to interactions among residents, among staff, and between residents and staff. When you enter an area, note how residents look and what they are doing.

Completion of the PAF gives you an ideal opportunity to rate the physical environment. For example, as you measure the hallways and rate the features available, also note their cleanliness, level of illumination, and the presence of odors. Then, as you complete the PAF sections on lounges and dining areas, rate these areas as well.

As you sit at the nurses' station or in a facility office tabulating information about the staff and residents, pay attention to the activities occurring around you; be particularly attentive to the noise level and the quality of staff-resident interactions.

Avoiding the Halo Effect

As you complete the Rating Scale, be aware of your overall impression, but do not let it affect the individual ratings of environmental characteristics. If the walls are newly painted, they should be rated "3" even if you do not like what is going on within them.

Your ratings should reflect your own assessments rather than staff or residents' views of the environment. Base your ratings on your direct observations and not on interviews with residents or conversations with staff.

Using the Full Range

Make your ratings so that for a given type of facility, the entire range (0-3) might potentially occur. In other words, the end points of the Rating Scale are defined as the best and worst conditions in that kind of facility. For ratings of some items, the same standard may not apply to different categories of facilities (e.g., congregate apartment housing and nursing homes). For most ratings, however, the same standards apply in different kinds of facilities.

There may be a tendency to give the benefit of the doubt when rating—to overlook or minimize negative aspects of the facility's condition. To counteract this tendency, if in doubt as to which of two ratings is appropriate, give the lower rating.

Environmental Variation

Environments vary in both time and space. For example, a dining hall may be quiet at 10:00 a.m. and noisy at 12:30 p.m. One bedroom may be fresh smelling, whereas another has unpleasant odors. Sample both kinds of variation: Observe more than one area of each type and at different times.

When making a composite rating in which you observe variability, consider several factors. First, the presence of variability generally precludes making a rating of 3; a 2 or 1 often signifies variability. Second, consider the overall prevalence of observations that merit the various ratings. If a particular observation occurs infrequently, your overall rating should be less affected by it. Third, in some cases a low rating overpowers the impressions gained at other times or in other areas. This is particularly the case for odors. For example, if one hallway is 0 on odors, the overall rating could be 0 even if other hallways are 2.

Scoring

Scoring can be done with the worksheets in Appendix B. Appendix C contains tables for transforming raw percentage scores into standard scores. Allow 20 minutes to score and profile the Rating Scale.

Specific Directions for the Rating Scale

Section I: Ratings of the Overall Site

Item 1: Neighborhood. Considering the facility's neighborhood as a place where you might live, how do you think the area around this site looks? Consider all factors that might influence your own selection of a neighborhood. Is there heavy traffic or loud industrial noise? Are the homes or businesses attractive and well maintained? Are the streets and sidewalks clean and free of litter?

Item 2: Grounds. Overall, how attractive are the site grounds? Take into account the season of the year and the extent of the grounds and landscaping. Note the presence of litter and weeds, the cleanliness and condition of parking lots and paths, and whether plants are trimmed around pathways. A rating of 2 implies that the grounds are landscaped or have very attractive natural vegetation and are well maintained. If a facility has no grounds or barren ground, rate this item 0.

Item 3: Buildings. How attractive are the site buildings? Evaluate not only the design but also the condition of the building. Note the condition of the roof, paint, and window trim; the state of the bricks, wood, or stucco; and any evidence of water stains and clogged gutters. Assign a rating of 1 to an ordinary, undecorated nursing home or apartment building. Poor maintenance reduces the rating of such a building to 0. Special decorative features raise the rating to a 2, whereas a 3 requires a unique and attractive design and excellent maintenance.

Section II, Ratings of Environmental Characteristics, Part I: Ratings of Four Major Living Areas

Some small facilities have no communal space for a lounge or dining room. Other facilities are designed to provide direct access to units from outside and may have no hallways—even in communal areas. If a facility has no space serving a particular function, leave those ratings blank. If an area is used for both lounging and dining, include ratings of this space under both categories.

Item 1: Noise Level. Make this rating only after sitting or working in an area for some time. Try to sample the area at different times during the day and during different functions. When you interview residents or talk to staff, note whether you have difficulty hearing or making yourself heard because of competing noises (e.g., shouting, loud TV, and cleaning equipment). As you work in an area, consider whether it is difficult to concentrate because of distractions. Listen for background noise such as traffic or music.

Item 2: Odors. Use your initial impressions to rate the presence of odors; otherwise, the rating may be inaccurate because of adaptation to pervasive odors. As noted previously, unpleasant odors, even if restricted to a few areas, will strongly weight the overall impression in a negative direction. Cooking odors may contribute to either a pleasant, fresh smell or to an unpleasant odor.

Item 3: Level of Illumination. Consider the illumination available from any source, natural or artificial. For the hallways, rate the illumination normally present. For the bedrooms, unoccupied rooms, or rooms in which residents can control the lighting, turn on the lights and then rate the illumination. Use a 3 if someone with impaired vision could read anywhere in the area. If a person could read, but only near a lamp or window, give a rating of 1. Clearly defined shadows or glare in some areas are clues to uneven illumination.

Items 4 and 5: Cleanliness and Condition. For floors and walls, it is sometimes difficult to determine when dirt has become part of the condition of the object. For example, a stain that cannot be removed from a rug is part of the rug's condition rather than its cleanliness. In general, any characteristic of an object that can be affected by a thorough cleaning is relevant to its cleanliness; any characteristic that cannot be affected by a thorough cleaning is relevant to its condition. Thus, scuff marks that could be washed off are considered soil, whereas marks where paint has been removed are considered damage.

Item 4: Cleanliness of Walls and Floors. To determine the cleanliness of walls, look particularly at the area around light switches, next to dining room tables or beds, and along handrails. On uncarpeted floors, stand so you can see light reflecting on the floor. Feel carpets or brush them with your hand to raise dirt that may be present. To merit a rating of 3, both walls and floors must be clean and free of scuff marks or fingerprints; the floors must be polished and the carpets free of dirt or debris and cleaned to remove spills. If these surfaces are cleaned regularly but are not spotless, give a rating of 2. If walls or floors (but not both) are poorly cleaned, give a rating of 1. If both walls and floors need a major cleaning (carpet infrequently or carelessly vacuumed and floors and walls dirty), rate them 0.

Item 5: Condition of Walls and Floors. Look for torn edges of linoleum, gouges in concrete, loose string or holes in carpets, cracks or warping in wood, faded or peeling paint, and cracks in plaster. Also consider what the surface would look like if thoroughly cleaned; surfaces that are in new condition should be rated so even if they are dirty. If walls, floors, or rugs need painting or replacement, rate them 0. If walls and floors look new, rate them 3.

Item 6: Condition of Furniture. Consider any burns, tears, or holes in upholstery; scratches, warping, or permanent stains on wood surfaces; loose seats, arms, or legs on chairs; and wobbly tables or chairs. Examine the surfaces for dirt, dust, stains, grime, spilled food, and ashes. Touch surfaces whenever possible. On wood surfaces, look for signs of polishing. On upholstered surfaces, look for stains and grime in the creases. A room rated 3 will show signs of regular dusting and polishing, and the upholstery will look new or regularly cleaned.

Item 7: Window Areas. Consider only the size and number of windows in relation to the size of the room; do not consider the view from the windows. Rate the windows with the curtains or drapes open, unless the windows are constantly covered, in which case they are functionally equivalent to having no windows at all.

Item 8: View From Windows. Section I includes ratings of the attractiveness of the neighborhood and of the grounds. Use Item 8 to rate the amount of stimulation available to a person looking out the windows. If the window is opaque or looks out onto a blank wall or empty alley, rate it 0. A window that overlooks a street merits a 2 or a 3. To rate a 3, the outside activity must be both varied and frequent. For example, human interactions on a playground are more variable than is traffic on a through street. A park may be frequently deserted or it may harbor nearly constant activity. Consider both variation and intensity of activity when making this rating.

Section II, Part II: Ratings of
Residents' Bedrooms or Apartments

These ratings apply only to the bedrooms or apartments and not to common areas.

Item 9: Variation in Design. To make this rating, think about whether you can identify individual rooms by their shape, size, color, furniture, and arrangement of furnishings. It may help to imagine that you are given photographs of each room. If the rooms vary so much that you would not know that they belong in the same building, then give a rating of 3. If you can easily distinguish individual rooms from the photographs, but can tell that they are all in the same building (common wall and floor coverings used, for example), rate this item 2. A 1 is appropriate where there are several distinct room types but where the rooms are very similar within one type. Rooms of a given type, however, must have some distinguishing details, such as different color schemes, to merit a 1. Rate this item 0 if rooms of a given type are indistinguishable or if rooms are identical except for decorative details (e.g., rug color or poster). In general, judge how easily someone with poor spatial orientation could tell his or her own room from someone else's.

Item 10: Personalization of Residents' Rooms (Apartments). Ratings on Items 9 and 10 are somewhat related. Insofar as people's personal belongings tend to be unique, rooms with more personalization will generally have greater variation in design. Variation in design, however, is possible without personalization of the room. You may need to ask residents if the furniture is their own. Note other details such as family photographs, books and magazines that are the resident's own, curtains, bedspreads, rugs, knickknacks, and the like.

Section II, Part III: Rating the Facility as a Whole

Item 11: Distinctiveness of Living Spaces. Included in this rating are residents' rooms (as a group) and all common areas but not spaces such as staff offices. In judging distinctiveness, consider furnishings, wall, and floor colors and texture; decorations such as pictures; windows; woodwork; and fixtures. For this rating, think of the impression the various areas would make if they were stripped of the furnishings that indicate the room's function. Could you tell the dining area from a bedroom or from the lounge (disregarding room size)? Consider how much the furniture adds to or counteracts this impression. Is the kind of furniture used quite similar, differing only in function (e.g., similar chairs in bedrooms, dining room, and lounge)? A 0 is applicable if floor and wall textures are quite similar, distinctive decorations are lacking, and the furnishings are quite similar in different areas.

Item 12: Overall Pleasantness of the Facility. Here is your opportunity to express your personal impressions of the facility. Make this rating as a summary of your experiences including your evaluation of interpersonal relations, the available resources, and the physical environment. Assume that the person being placed requires the level of care provided by the facility.

Item 13: Overall Attractiveness of the Facility. This item summarizes your aesthetic impression of the facility. This personal judgment combines impressions of the cleanliness, condition, and style of decor. Include the furniture, draperies, carpets, paintings, plants, flowers, color scheme, woodwork, walls, and so on.

Section III: Ratings of Residents

In these ratings, include only those residents in the common living areas; do not include people who are in their own rooms. Where you see great variation between individuals, note it, but make one rating of the overall impression. If a substantial minority fall into a lower rating, give the lower rating to the whole.

Item 1: Personal Grooming. As you interview residents and observe them in the common areas, rate their cleanliness; the condition of their hair, nails, and so on; and whether the men are shaven. Unpleasant odors emanating from individual residents merit a rating of 0. Do not include clothing in this rating.

Item 2: Condition of Clothing. Do not rate style, only condition.

Item 3: Interaction of Residents. Try to observe residents in a variety of situations such as during mealtimes, activities, and free time. Do residents talk to each other when they sit together at meals? Do they leave as soon as the meal or activity is over or do they prolong the period of contact? When free to be with others or not, do residents interact with each other?

Item 4: Brief Verbal Exchanges. Here again, observe residents in various situations such as at meals, passing each other in the hall, or joining an activity.

Item 5: General Amount of Activity. Because a variety of behaviors qualify as activity for Item 5, you need to exercise a good deal of judgment. Count as an activity any behavior that seems purposeful even if it is sedentary. Thus, socializing with others, reading, or watching TV or an ongoing activity is considered activity, whereas wandering, staring blankly, or dozing is not.

Section IV: Ratings of Staff

Always be alert to the ways in which staff members interact with residents and with each other. As with all ratings, try to sample a variety of situations involving not only job-related contacts but informal contacts as well. For example, note how the administrator, activity director, and other staff address residents in a meeting and in passing them in the hall. Try to observe unobtrusively (e.g., when you are tabulating information) so you can ascertain the quality of interactions when participants are not "on stage" for an outside observer.

Item 1: Quality of Interaction. This item includes descriptors of the quality of interaction between staff and residents. Base your rating on direct observation and on attitudes that staff members may express to you (e.g., condescension).

Item 2: Physical Contact With Residents. Observe various staff members in their interactions with residents; rate the general tone of the physical contact.

Item 3: Organization. During your interactions with the administrator, staff members, and residents, note how efficiently procedures are organized and residents' needs are handled. Does the administrator seem to be on top of conditions within the facility? Some indicators of effective organization are the ability to locate information readily, being knowledgeable about who handles specific responsibilities within the facility, and clarity in answering questions about the functioning of the facility. Also note whether nursing and personal care services are provided on time and efficiently. Are meal trays delivered quickly and to the right person? Are medications given efficiently and on time? Do residents have to wait unduly long to get up in the morning, to be bathed, or to be taken to activities?

Item 4: Availability of Staff to Residents. Be alert to staff presence, particularly in the halls and in the rooms or apartments. For example, observe whether staff members visit residents in their rooms and, if so, for what purpose. When you leave a resident's room, note how far you would need to go to find a staff member. Also make note of instances of residents' needs going unattended or of residents relying on one another or outsiders for assistance. Finally, inquire of staff members whether residents are observed or checked in a regular or scheduled manner.

To rate a 3, a nursing station or staff office must be in view of all rooms and must be generally occupied. A 2 is appropriate if checks on each resident are scheduled and systematic. A 1 indicates that observation is somewhat haphazard and that a resident might search for some time before finding a staff member. A rating of 0 is appropriate when staff-resident contacts occur irregularly, are secondary results of other activities, and are usually initiated by residents.

Item 5: Staff Conflict. Because staff will normally minimize open conflict in the presence of outsiders, you must be alert to subtle signs of discord. Your rating should reflect any hint of conflict you see because it probably indicates strong underlying feelings.

8

RESEARCH APPLICATIONS
AND FINDINGS

Investigators have used the Multiphasic Environmental Assessment Procedure (MEAP) to differentiate types of facilities, to study the multidimensional nature of quality of care, and to focus on the compatibility of high-quality care and for-profit ownership. They have also examined how physical features and program policies alter the social climate of a facility, how social climate factors are related to residents' activity levels and community contact, and how relocation affects long-term care residents. The results of research with the MEAP have been published in more than 150 journal articles and reports.

This chapter covers some of the important research applications of the MEAP including its use to describe and compare facilities, to conceptualize the program environment as a system, and to measure program impact.

DESCRIBING AND
COMPARING FACILITIES

We designed the MEAP to describe and compare varied types of residential programs for older adults. The MEAP has been adapted for similar uses in other countries and in other types of residential and nonresidential programs.

Residential Programs for Older Adults

Comparisons Among Programs. Billingsley and Batterson (1986) used the MEAP to evaluate a group of facilities administered by a nonprofit agency. Administrators used the findings to discuss facility development with advisory committees, conduct staff development workshops, and meet with residents' councils to plan policy and program changes. Feedback to managers and staff helped them understand their facility and examine whether it was accomplishing its goals.

Even within the same organization, facilities may target different subgroups of the elderly population. Thus, compared with its market-rate apartments, the subsidized apartments run by this nonprofit corporation served a population with fewer social resources, indicating that they were meeting one of their program goals. On the other hand, some patterns of Sheltered Care Environment Scale (SCES) results were consistent across all the facilities and were thought to reflect the corporation's philosophy and management style.

To help characterize the program provided by different types of long-term care, Braun and Rose (1989) used portions of the Policy and Program Information Form (POLIF) to assess skilled nursing facilities, intermediate care facilities, foster homes, a day hospital, and comprehensive home care. The foster care and day hospital programs had the highest expectations of patient functioning, followed by intermediate care and skilled nursing facilities. The home care settings were the most accepting of patient disabilities and problem behaviors. Somewhat unexpectedly, however, intermediate care and skilled nursing facilities were less accepting of problem behavior than was the day hospital and no more accepting than were foster homes. In general, skilled nursing facilities and home care programs were able to provide the most nursing services and thus to manage the most impaired patients.

Formal and informal care settings were also compared by Perkins, King, and Hollyman (1989), who used adapted versions of the Physical and Architectural Features Checklist (PAF) and POLIF to assess a group of small, private homes for community placement of older psychiatric patients in Great Britain. Compared with public residential care homes, the private homes were higher on privacy, choice, encouragement of resident autonomy, and resident involvement in the organization of home life. In addition, these private homes were higher on physical amenities and safety features but lower on prosthetic, orientational, and social-recreational aids. The relative lack of supportive physical features may reflect the more homelike style of the private homes, which therefore may not be suitable for very impaired residents. Overall, residents were at least as satisfied with their lives in these homes as they had been with their lives in the hospital. Moreover, residents' behavioral problems, apathy, and physical disability decreased after placement from the hospital to the private homes.

Sewell and colleagues (Sewell & Lethaby, 1990; Sewell & Marquis, 1989) used the PAF, POLIF, and parts of the Resident and Staff Information Form (RESIF) to assess a sample of 183 residential and 87 hospital units in New Zealand and found that the various types of facilities differed in some expected ways. For example, resident functional abilities and activity level, as well as rated resident functioning, were higher in intermediate care units than in long-term care units (Sewell & Marquis, 1989). The PAF showed that the intermediate care units had more physical amenities; raters also saw them as more attractive.

In addition, residential homes offered fewer supportive features and medical services but more opportunities for resident choice and control than did hospital units (Sewell & Lethaby, 1990). Other researchers have found similar differences between hospital- and community-based settings for the elderly. For example, Benjamin and Spector (1990) and Philp, Mutch, Devaney, and Ogston (1989) found that British nursing homes and residential care facilities provided more privacy, choice, and resident control than did long-term care hospital units.

Cross-Cultural Adaptations. The MEAP has been used extensively in English-speaking countries other than the United States including Australia (Manning, 1989), Canada (Hodge, 1987), Great Britain (Benjamin & Spector, 1990, 1992; Netten, 1992), and New Zealand (Sewell & Lethaby, 1990; Sewell & Marquis, 1989). In addition, the MEAP has been translated and adapted for use in a number of countries: Denmark (Ramian, 1987), Japan (Kodama, 1986, 1988a, 1988b), The Netherlands (Peters & Boerma, 1982, 1983; van Weert & Beuken, 1987), Spain (Izal, 1992), and Sweden (Svensson, 1984).

Some cross-cultural applications of the MEAP have focused on how facilities in other countries compare with the norms obtained in the United States. Compared with American nursing home norms, for example, Netten (1992) found that staff in British homes rated them lower on cohesion, independence, and organization and higher on conflict and resident influence. Residents in these homes were older but somewhat higher functioning than American nursing home residents.

Fernandez-Ballesteros and colleagues (1991) applied a Spanish adaptation of the MEAP to 32 residential care facilities. They found that Spanish residential care facilities were generally comparable to American facilities in the characteristics of their residents and staff. With the exception of fewer amenities and safety features, they also had similar physical features. Their policies and services differed in that they were more accepting of problem behavior, had fewer formal procedures for communicating with residents and staff, and provided more health services. Outside observers rated Spanish facilities somewhat lower than American facilities on all four of the Rating Scale subscales. Finally, residents and staff in the Spanish facilities reported less cohesion, organization, and physical comfort and more conflict. In addition, residents reported more self-disclosure in the Spanish facilities. According to the authors, some of these findings may reflect differences between the Spanish and American social context; for example, Spaniards may be more critical and expressive (high self-disclosure and conflict and low physical comfort).

Data from these facilities were used to examine the psychometrics of the Spanish MEAP. Despite the homogeneity of the sample (all facilities were residential care type), individual items showed reasonable response distributions. As might be expected from the greater homogeneity of the sample, the internal consistencies of the Spanish MEAP subscales were somewhat lower than those of the American version. The subscale intercorrelations were roughly comparable to those obtained in the American normative sample. Interjudge reliability on the POLIF subscales was moderate to high; as was the agreement between residents and staff and between different groups of residents on the SCES subscales. Interjudge reliability on the Rating Scale was also acceptable (Izal, 1992).

Applications to Psychiatric Settings

Researchers have applied the MEAP to psychiatric settings. For example, Manning (1989) used the MEAP to assess Australian Richmond Fellowship Homes, which are halfway houses for adults with psychiatric disorders. As expected from their adherence to a therapeutic community model, these homes were high on resident choice and control. On the other hand, they provided few health services. Except for orientational aids and facilities for staff, the homes had most of the physical features found in the U.S. normative sample. Despite their common model of treatment, the RESIF pointed to differences between homes in their resident characteristics—differences that may be related to treatment outcome.

Garritson (1987) compared locked and unlocked psychiatric units by having nurses complete parts of the POLIF. As expected, locked psychiatric units had less resident control than did unlocked units; locked and unlocked units, however, did not differ in terms of their acceptance of problem behavior. Garritson concluded that patients who are admitted voluntarily and are thus capable of making decisions should be placed in unlocked wards in which they have more such opportunities. Nearly half the patients in the locked units in Garritson's study were voluntary admissions.

Using the MEAP as a model, Timko (1995) developed the Residential Substance Abuse and Psychiatric Programs Inventory (RESPPI). Normative data are available from 96 representative programs. Comparisons between program types indicate that substance abuse programs demanded higher functioning, were less tolerant of problem behavior, provided less choice and privacy, had more structures for resident involvement and communication, and provided fewer daily living services than did general psychiatric programs (Timko, 1995).

Hospital-Based and Community-Based Treatment. In an effort to understand the alternatives to institutionalization, a number of researchers have used the MEAP to compare hospital-based treatment within community-based group homes. In general, hospital settings provide more services and physical resources in a more restrictive environment. For example, using the RESPPI, Timko (1995) found that community-based substance abuse programs had higher expectations regarding resident functional independence, provided residents more choice and control, and provided fewer services than did hospital-based substance abuse programs. Compared with community-based programs, hospital programs had more social-recreational and prosthetic aids, safety features, staff facilities, and space (Timko, in press).

Lehman, Possidente, and Hawker (1986) examined the quality of life experienced by chronically mentally ill persons who lived either in a state hospital or in supervised community residences. Compared with hospitalized patients, community residents described their living situations as more cohesive and comfortable and more oriented toward independence and resident influence. As expected, community residents were more satisfied with their living situation than were patients in the hospital (see also Lehman, 1988).

Similarly, Maloney and Bowman (1982) found that residents and staff agreed that group homes were higher on cohesion, independence, organization, and physical comfort and lower on conflict than the hospital unit from which patients were placed. Residents and staff in the group homes also showed closer agreement on the social climate than did residents and staff in the hospital unit. As expected, acceptance of problem behavior was higher in the hospital setting.

Linn and colleagues (1985) followed long-term, mentally ill men who were referred for nursing home placement from eight Veterans Administration (VA) medical centers. The MEAP was used to assess the community nursing homes, VA nursing care units, and VA psychiatric wards to which they were referred. Compared with VA psychiatric units, the community nursing homes had more functionally impaired residents, fewer staff resources, and less restrictive policies. VA nursing care units were midway between community nursing homes and VA psychiatric units in their policies and similar to the other VA units in the characteristics of their residents and staff (Timko, Nguyen, Williford, & Moos, 1993).

Nelson and Earls (1986) studied the housing quality of psychiatric patients who had been discharged into the community. They used the MEAP Rating Scale to help develop a measure of clients' perceptions of the quality of their community housing. Many of the clients reported concerns about their housing such as noise level, odor, poor quality of lighting, poor condition of walls and floors, and lack of adequate windows. Clients who roomed in a private home or boarding home reported twice as many concerns about their housing as did those who lived in their own homes, in their parents' homes, or in a supervised group home. About 15% of the clients reported seven or more concerns about their housing such as high noise level, foul odors, poor quality of lighting, poor condition of walls and floors, and lack of adequate windows.

Adaptations to Other Settings

The MEAP has been adapted for use in residential facilities for developmentally disabled people and for problem youth, as well as in adult day care and inpatient hospital units.

Residential Settings for Developmentally Disabled Persons. To help developmentally disabled persons respond to the SCES, Wadsworth and

Harper (1988) constructed a picture-prompted version of three of the subscales (Cohesion, Conflict, and Independence). The 1-week and 6-week test-retest reliabilities of the picture-cued questions were higher than those for the verbal items only. The addition of picture cues can help increase the reliability of residential evaluations obtained from moderately mentally retarded persons (Wadsworth & Harper, 1989). In another application, Campbell and Bailey (1984) drew on MEAP items to develop an inventory to assess and classify community residential settings for mentally disabled persons. (For a discussion of the application of the MEAP to residential settings for developmentally disabled persons, see Wandersman & Moos, 1981a, 1981b.)

Families of developmentally disabled clients seem to play a much larger role in advocacy efforts than do relatives of mentally ill clients. To see whether such advocacy efforts are associated with differences in the quality of group homes for these populations, Wilson and Kouzi (1990) compared 238 group homes for mentally disabled clients with 159 homes for developmentally disabled clients. Overall, facilities for developmentally disabled clients offered more assistance with personal care and daily living tasks. These facilities were also smaller and had better trained staff. Facilities for developmentally disabled clients scored higher on a summary of 32 environmental factors from the Rating Scale as well as on global comfort, personalization, and resident-staff interaction.

Older individuals may require supportive environmental features that may contribute to making the facility seem more institutional. Compared with a facility for young adults, Rovins (1990) found that a residential facility for older, mentally disabled adults had more prosthetic aids but lacked personalization and was less homelike with respect to community accessibility and bedroom and bathroom design. Thus, a key challenge is to structure environments that meet older adults' needs for care and medical treatment without making them more impersonal.

Residential Settings for Problem Youth. An adaptation of the MEAP was used to evaluate community-based residential facilities for troubled youth including secure detention facilities, nonsecure alternatives to detention such as emergency shelters, group homes, and residential treatment (Linney, 1982). It provided useful information regarding the extent of normalization in these settings and distinguished among these programs. Observers' impressions about the pleasantness and variety of the physical environment and the resident and staff functioning, as measured by the Rating Scale, were related in expected ways to organizational control and program design measures (Mulvey, Linney, & Rosenberg, 1987).

Adult Day Care Settings. Several researchers have used the conceptual framework underlying the MEAP and adapted the MEAP items to measure the quality of adult day care programs. For example, Lyman (1990) used the PAF and POLIF as guides to compare 2-day care programs and understand the sources of staff work stress.

In an extended program of research, Conrad, Hanrahan, and Hughes (1988) constructed the Adult Day Care Assessment Procedure, which measures characteristics of the client population, provision of services and activities, and the quality of the social environment. Findings on more than 900 day care programs showed that a high proportion of the clients had moderate to severe impairments in activities of daily living and that, overall, the programs were characterized by complex and somewhat fragmented policies (Conrad, Hanrahan, & Hughes, 1990; Conrad & Miller, 1987). Such information can help in formulating quality standards for adult day care programs.

Some day care programs specialize in serving clients with Alzheimer's disease. Compared with non-Alzheimer's programs, these programs provided more case management, health evaluation, training in activities of daily living, therapeutic activity, and family involvement (Conrad et al., 1988; Conrad, Hughes, Hanrahan, & Wang, 1993). Thus, the two sets of programs provided services and activities that were generally consistent with their clients' pattern of impairment. The ability to make valid characterizations of models of programs and their intended clients enables practitioners to match patients with appropriate health care settings.

In a similar effort, Weissert and colleagues (1989) adapted the PAF to explore the relationships between client attributes, staff resources, services and other program resources, and client satisfaction in three types of day care programs: nursing home-rehabilitation hospital, general hospital-social service agency, and special-purpose programs. Nursing home-rehabilitation hospital centers were more likely to have physical therapy and bathing facilities, consistent with their location in inpatient facilities. Otherwise, however, there were few differences among the three models in their physical facilities and equipment. Given that the patient populations in these three models differed significantly, these findings imply some mismatch between patients' needs and available physical resources.

Medical Units. Porter and Watson (1985) used the MEAP Rating Scale to assess 24 inpatient medical units on five occasions over a period of several years. One unit and its grounds were renovated during the study period, and the effects were reflected in increased physical attractiveness scores. Environmental diversity was especially low in the intensive care units, although one unit improved over an 18-month period as patients personalized their rooms by displaying pictures and cards on the bulletin boards and bedside tables.

With respect to medical treatment outcome, Oberle, Wry, and Paul (1988) found that the improved physical amenities and security features in a new hospital building were associated with lower anxiety and less use of pain-control medications among postoperative surgery patients. Concomitant changes in service provision and staff morale and job performance may also have affected patients' outcomes.

Developing Program Models

Various typologies have been proposed for classifying residential programs. Typologies facilitate discussion and analysis by reducing the amount of detail. For example, we conducted an empirical cluster analysis of SCES data from 235 programs and identified six distinct clusters of facilities (Timko & Moos, 1991b).

Supportive, self-directed facilities are characterized by high scores on cohesion, independence, and resident influence and low scores on conflict. Thus, these facilities emphasize harmonious relationships and resident autonomy. These facilities are also well organized and comfortable. Residents in these facilities tend to keep their personal feelings and concerns to themselves. Supportive, well-organized facilities also emphasize harmonious interpersonal relationships and independence, although not as strongly as the first cluster. Facilities in this cluster are well organized and comfortable, but the emphasis on resident influence is much lower.

Open conflict facilities are characterized by conflict; residents openly share their personal problems and their angry and critical feelings about each other and the facility. They do so in the absence of warm, intimate relationships and comfortable surroundings. This facility type displays below-average emphasis on cohesion, organization, and physical comfort. Suppressed conflict facilities are below average on all subscales except Conflict, which is moderately emphasized. Although residents are angry and critical, they tend to keep their personal feelings to themselves.

Emergent-positive facilities are average or above average on all seven subscales. The strongest characteristic of the social climate in emergent-positive facilities is the emphasis on resident influence. In contrast with supportive, self-directed settings, however, residents are critical, outspoken, and self-revealing. Unresponsive facilities are average or below average on all seven subscales. In particular, unresponsive facilities lack emphasis on aspects of social climate that reflect responsiveness to residents' preferences and needs. Little emphasis is placed on independence, self-disclosure, or resident influence. The facility may provide adequate care, but residents are disengaged and passive.

Facilities that provide less care and nonprofit and larger facilities were more likely to be of the supportive types. Facilities housing more socially competent and women residents were more likely to be of the supportive, self-directed type. The type of social climate was also related to resident adaptation. Residents in the supportive types of facilities were seen by observers as better functioning, were more involved in self-initiated activities, and used fewer health services (Timko & Moos, 1991b).

In a cluster analysis of SCES data from British group homes, Netten (1991-1992, 1992) classified British group homes in terms of their type of regime (positive, mixed, and restrictive). Positive homes were high on SCES cohesion, independence, organization, self-disclosure, and resident influence. Mixed homes were higher than restrictive homes on independence and resident influence. Regimes classified as positive were associated with better outcomes for cognitively impaired residents.

Overall, a configurational approach to describing social climate and other aspects of group-living settings may help to develop specific program models and to place individual residents in the most appropriate housing.

CONCEPTUALIZING THE PROGRAM
ENVIRONMENT AS A SYSTEM

A facility's environment is a system of interrelated factors. We formulated a model of the residential program as a dynamic system composed of the institutional context (factors such as ownership and size) and four sets of variables: aggregate resident and staff characteristics, physical features, policies and services, and social climate (see Figure 8.1). The model posits that ownership and size are associated with the aggregate characteristics of the residents and staff in a facility; in turn, aggregate resident and staff characteristics are associated with the physical features,

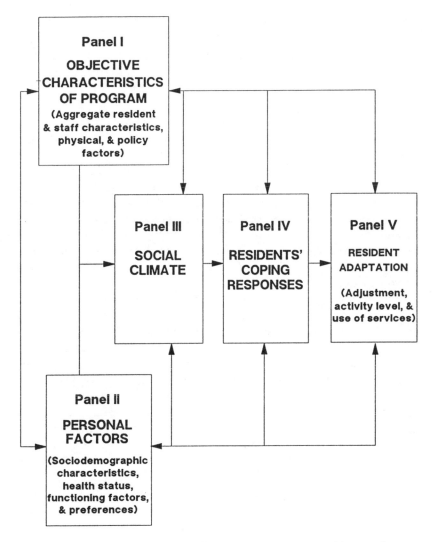

Figure 8.1. A Model of the Relationship Between Program and Personal Factors and Resident Adaptation

policies, and services in the facility. Together, these factors help determine the facility's social climate.

The MEAP can help to clarify how these factors relate to each other. For example, research with the MEAP has focused on such issues as how nonprofit facilities differ from proprietary facilities, how facility size affects services and policies, and how the physical resources in a facility are related to its resident population and policies.

Institutional Context

Ownership. In the normative sample, we found that nonprofit facilities had more physical resources (especially physical amenities, social-recreational aids, and space for residents and staff) and more resident-oriented policies (acceptance of problem behavior, provision for privacy and resident control, and health services). Nonprofit facilities also tended to be seen by residents as more cohesive and well organized, more oriented toward resident self-direction, and more physically comfortable than were proprietary facilities. Some of these advantages of nonprofit ownership appeared to be stronger for residential care facilities than for apartments and nursing homes (Lemke & Moos, 1986, 1989a; Moos & Lemke, 1980).

Like nonprofit facilities, veterans facilities provide more physical resources than do proprietary settings. Specifically, veterans facilities had more physical amenities and social-recreational aids, as well as more space for resident functions, than did proprietary facilities. In contrast, veterans facilities had fewer safety features and were less accessible to community resources than either the proprietary or the nonprofit facilities. These differences generally held for both nursing home and residential care (domiciliary) facilities. They reflect the age of the buildings that house many of the veterans facilities, the more generous space allowances typically made in older buildings, and their location in full-service medical centers and consequent isolation from community resources.

For veterans facilities, public ownership was related to high levels of service and a more bureaucratic and structured organization. As a consequence of their location in full-service medical centers, veterans facilities offered a greater diversity of services than did either proprietary or nonprofit facilities. Veterans facilities, however, provided their residents less privacy, less flexibility in organizing their daily lives, and less input into facility governance. We also found that both residents and staff in veterans facilities reported less warmth and self-direction than did residents and staff in proprietary or private nonprofit facilities. These differences held after matching facilities by size and resident functional ability (Lemke & Moos, 1989a; Moos & Lemke, 1994).

In general, these results are consistent with prior research and with intuitive expectations about the differences between ownership types. The findings confirm the superiority of nonprofit facilities, particularly in areas that are more difficult to regulate such as the comfort of the physical environment and the quality of the social environment. They also show that veterans facilities tend to provide high-quality care but that they are somewhat regimented and have a less cohesive social climate.

Size. Compared with smaller community facilities, larger community facilities enjoy a number of advantages in terms of their physical features and services. In the normative sample, larger facilities had more physical amenities, supportive features, and space for staff functions but somewhat less space for residents. These relationships were somewhat stronger in proprietary than in nonprofit facilities.

Larger community facilities also offered more health services and social-recreational activities and had a more diverse and experienced staff. In addition, larger facilities had policies that provide more opportunities for personal control—specifically, more choice in daily routines, more resident control, and more privacy. Larger facilities were also more likely to institute procedures for systematically communicating policies to residents and staff. These findings run counter to the idea that large size necessarily leads to a more restrictive environment. The more formal organizational structure and service provision in large facilities, however, may contribute to their more bureaucratic feel. In contrast with the pattern for physical features, these findings applied more strongly in nonprofit than in proprietary facilities (Lemke & Moos, 1986).

Finally, residents in larger facilities reported more emphasis on independence but also poorer organization and more conflict (Lemke & Moos, 1980, 1986; Moos & Lemke, 1994). Large institutions may be more impersonal, discordant, and chaotic due to their somewhat more crowded conditions and more complex social structure. The sheer number of residents and staff and the increased hierarchy of large institutions may make communication more difficult, but these factors may also encourage a greater emphasis on having residents do as much as they can for themselves. Large facility size may reduce pressure to conform and to suppress anger. As evidence, we found that residents also report more self-disclosure in larger facilities.

Overall, larger facilities are able to provide a wider array of physical features and services and need not develop a more bureaucratic and restrictive environment, although they are somewhat more chaotic and evidence more interpersonal conflict.

Resident Selection and Allocation

We have found wide variations in the characteristics of residents in different types of facilities. These differences reflect the operation of mechanisms of self-selection and social allocation that determine where a person is likely to live. Research with the MEAP has identified two distinct resident-facility matching processes. One process is guided by residents' functional ability and need for services; the other reflects predisposing and enabling factors that make it possible for more privileged residents to live together and obtain access to richer physical resources and services. (For more details, see Lemke & Moos, 1981; Moos & Lemke, 1994.)

Selection Into Different Levels of Care. Functional ability, one main index of need for services, is an important selection criterion into long-term care and into different levels of care. As noted previously, we found marked differences in the current functioning of residents in the three levels of care. These findings indicate a relatively good match of older people's functional and health status to different levels of residential services.

Thus, for example, more impaired residents, who are more likely to live in nursing homes, have more prosthetic aids and access to more services but are given fewer opportunities for choice, control, and privacy. Moderately impaired residents, who are more likely to live in residential care facilities, have somewhat higher levels of privacy and lower levels of services. Apartment residents have access to fewer services in the facility but exercise more choice and control, enjoy more privacy, and can more easily access community resources.

Need factors have the most important impact on the type of facility entered, but once need is taken into account predisposing and enabling factors have moderate effects. We found that residents in the three sets of community facilities were drawn from roughly comparable social backgrounds, although nursing home residents were less well educated, of lower occupational status, and more likely to be receiving public assistance than were residents in the other two types of facilities. In general, social and financial resources help older people remain in lower levels of care.

Selection Into Specific Facilities Within Levels of Care. In addition to differences in the resident populations of facilities that provide different levels of care, facilities of a given level of care show substantial variations as well. Functional impairment and need for services, which form the major basis for selection of an appropriate level of care, are less important in the choice of facilities within each level. After level of care is controlled, residents whose functioning was more impaired were in less spacious facilities and had access to fewer social-recreational aids. Moreover, except for prosthetic aids, impaired residents did not have access to more supportive physical features. Residents who were more impaired tended to be in facilities that provided less daily living assistance and no more health services, even though these facilities had lower expectations for functioning. These residents also had less policy choice, resident control, and privacy.

Education, socioeconomic status, and other selection factors affect the likelihood of placement in a particular setting, thus increasing the homogeneity of a facility's residents and giving facilities distinctive character. In the normative group, older people who had better personal resources were more likely to live in residential settings with more physical resources, more flexible policies, more services, more staff, and better-qualified staff. After level of care was controlled, social status characteristics were as closely related to the physical features, policies, and services available to residents as were residents' functional abilities. These findings show that enabling factors make a difference in the resources available in old age.

Relationships Among Program Characteristics

Physical Features, Policies, and Services. In general, better physical features are associated with more resident-directed policies and the provision of more services. In the normative sample, we found that facilities with more social-recreational, prosthetic, and orientational aids and more space for staff functions provided their residents with more privacy, more choice in daily life, and more say in facility governance (Moos, 1981; Moos & Lemke, 1980, 1994). In addition, facilities with more social-recreational aids tended to be higher on choice and control and those with better access to community resources tended to offer their residents more choice.

Determinants of Social Climate. Why do residential environments develop in such disparate ways? What leads to an emphasis on cohesion, independence, or order? How does a particular social climate evolve from the discrete features and people that constitute the setting? To what extent do physical and policy factors influence the social climate that develops in a residential facility?

In a sample of 244 community facilities, we found that residents reported more interpersonal support and resident self-direction (higher independence and resident influence) in facilities with more physical resources and with policies providing more resident control, privacy, policy clarity, and social-recreational activities; there was a similar pattern for staff's perceptions of resident self-direction. More privacy was also associated with better organization and less conflict. Facilities in which residents had more social resources were seen by residents and staff as providing more interpersonal support, resident self-direction, and organization. These findings, which reflect predictable associations between physical, policy, and suprapersonal factors and the social climate in a facility, may help to improve residential facilities by suggesting factors that can be targeted in interventions (Moos & Lemke, 1994; Timko & Moos, 1990).

THE IMPACT OF RESIDENTIAL PROGRAMS

The MEAP has been used in summative evaluation studies in which the subscales are related to outcome criteria such as resident morale and well-being. For example, a facility's policy and social climate resources may influence residents' activity levels, satisfaction, and morbidity. Moreover, any such impacts may vary for residents depending on factors such as their functional abilities. These issues can be examined at the facility and individual levels of analysis using the framework summarized in Figure 8.1 (see also Moos & Lemke, 1985, 1994).

The Residential Environment and Group Outcomes

At the group level of analysis, we noted that policies, such as resident control of decision making, and aspects of program social climate, such as independence and resident influence, were associated with residents' involvement in activities in the community (David, Moos, & Kahn, 1981). We found that facilities with policies that allow more privacy, choice, and control, and whose social climates were more oriented toward independence and resident influence, tended to have residents who were rated as higher functioning, who were more involved in self-initiated activities in the community, and who used fewer health and daily living services (Moos & Lemke, 1994; Timko & Moos, 1989).

We also found some important congruence effects (Moos & Lemke, 1994). In general, policies that provide more personal control are more closely associated with well-being and use of services among functionally intact than among functionally impaired resident groups. Specifically, more policy choice and an independence-oriented social climate were associated with less use of facility health and daily living services among better-functioning resident groups. These facility characteristics were not associated with use of services among more impaired resident groups. Overall, these findings are consistent with the idea that policies that provide more choice and control are particularly important for groups of relatively intact residents; these factors may be less salient for groups of impaired residents.

Staff Morale and Turnover. According to Willcocks, Peace, and Kellaher (1987), staff may pay a price for policies that focus too much on resident needs. Residents and staff in 100 British residential homes completed questionnaires covering their morale and well-being. Staff tended to be less anxious and more satisfied with their jobs when their needs for resident safety, security, and structure were met. Staff reported more worries in homes that had more resident-oriented policies.

In nursing homes, social climate, physical design, and staff turnover may be linked. Specifically, we found that staff turnover was higher in community facilities in which staff reported more conflict and less cohesion, organization, and resident influence (Brennan & Moos, 1990). Efforts to reduce conflict and encourage mutual helping among staff and residents may lead to improved employee retention.

In veterans facilities, there was more staff turnover when organization was high and resident influence was low; facilities such as these may be somewhat rigid, overly structured workplaces that demoralize staff. Staff turnover was also high when organization was low and resident influence was high. A poorly organized facility in which residents have considerable influence may be chaotic for staff and may lack clear and consistent guidelines for resident and staff conduct. Such a facility may promote staff turnover because it caters more to residents' than staff's needs.

The Residential Environment and Individual Outcomes

The links between the residential environment and outcomes have also been examined in terms of the individual resident's functioning and well-being.

Activity Involvement. At the individual level of analysis, we found that provisions for privacy and policies oriented toward personal control were associated with greater involvement in self-initiated activities in the facility and in the community and less participation in facility-sponsored activities (Lemke & Moos, 1989b). Residents of facilities that were seen as friendly, well organized, and oriented toward independence and resident influence were also more likely to participate in self-initiated activities. (For a study focused on group homes for psychiatric clients, see Manning, 1989.)

We also identified some person-environment congruence effects with respect to residents' involvement in both self-initiated and facility-sponsored activities. A number of facility features had a strong positive relationship to self-initiated activity for residents with intact functioning, a somewhat positive relationship for moderately impaired residents, and either a weak positive or no relationship for residents with severe impairment. For example, high-functioning residents initiated more activity in settings in which other residents had more social resources and were more functionally able and more active, in which policies promoted more personal control, in which there were more cohesion and organization, and in which residents saw the facility as oriented more toward self-direction. These environmental factors seem to operate as a stimulus to independent activity for residents who are relatively intact or only moderately impaired.

Our findings were somewhat different for residents' participation in facility-sponsored activities. Residents were more likely to participate in facility activities in settings with less privacy, choice, and control. Thus, a high level of participation in facility activities may be one part of a policy orientation toward making decisions for residents and encouraging group participation. In general, these results are consistent with our earlier findings that groups of residents in facilities low on personal control policies are more likely to use the available facility services.

As with self-initiated activities, residents' functional abilities moderated the association between facility features and residents' participation in planned activities. For example, for relatively independent residents the level of personal control policies was not related to their participation in planned activities. In contrast, more impaired residents were less likely to participate in planned activities in facilities high on resident choice and control (Lemke & Moos, 1989b; Moos & Lemke, 1994).

Together with other research, our findings also suggest that facility size operates as an environmental demand. Specifically, functional ability moderated the influence of size on residents' participation in planned activities. In large facilities, functionally able residents are somewhat more involved in facility-organized activities than are impaired residents. As size decreases, these group differences become smaller; in fact, in small facilities more impaired residents were more involved in planned activities. These findings suggest that large facilities may exceed the level of demand that is optimal for impaired residents and that small facilities may fail to provide sufficient challenge and range of choice for intact older people (Lemke & Moos, 1989b).

Mood and Satisfaction. A number of researchers have examined environmental factors that predict individual residents' mood and satisfaction. For example, Thomas (1989) followed older people who were newly admitted to long-term care residences. Those residents who moved into settings in which interpersonal rapport was higher and residents had more autonomy were more satisfied at the end of 9 months. Phillips and Henderson (1991) also found a relationship between the social environment and residents' mood; residents were more likely to have depressive symptoms in nursing homes that staff saw as low on cohesion, self-disclosure, and resident influence.

Kruzich, Clinton, and Kelber (1992) found that environmental diversity and physical attractiveness of the unit were related to greater satisfaction among cognitively competent nursing home residents. They found evidence of congruence effects: Physical attractiveness was more important for physically impaired residents, whereas environmental diversity was more important for more intact residents. Greater resident involvement in decision making was related to lower satisfaction with the nursing home but only among the physically more dependent residents.

Predictors of Mortality. Braun (1991) followed a group of veterans discharged to nursing homes. The nursing homes were assessed with the MEAP, and a quality index was constructed (basically the average of the quality indices described in Chapter 1 and the four Rating Scale dimensions). In conjunction with registered nurse hours and a measure of the process of care, higher scores on the quality index were related to less than expected mortality over the 6-month follow-up. The PAF index of security was most closely related to lower mortality. The provision of physical features that support optimum functioning may serve as a proxy for overall nursing home quality and may reflect a commitment of the administration to prevent disorientation, increase adaptation to functional limitations, and protect residents' welfare.

Relocation and Residents' Behavior and Use of Space. As noted previously, the PAF can help to specify changes in the physical environment when residents are relocated. In such a study, we conceptualized changes in behavior as attempts to adapt to the larger design and altered layout of a new building, in particular, to the separation of caregiving and social spaces (Moos, David, Lemke, & Postle, 1984). The new building provided more physical amenities and prosthetic features, fewer orientational aids, a more complex floor plan, and increased distance between the social areas and nurses' stations. The new building had a different pattern of use: The hallways adjacent to the nurse's stations were used as lounges by residents who were trying to maintain contact with staff activity, and the special activity areas drew increased use because of the conjunction of well-furnished spaces and program changes.

We used a model of person-environment congruence to try to explain the impact of the relocation on the behavior of residents who varied in mobility and mental status. Improved accessibility in the new facility benefited wheelchair-mobile residents, but immobile residents experienced less stimulation and restriction of their spatial range as a result of the dispersion of functional spaces. High mental status residents were drawn out of their bedrooms into social spaces, whereas low mental status residents spent less time in social areas and more in the halls near the nurses' stations where they could maintain contact with staff (Lemke & Moos, 1984).

Psychiatric Treatment Outcome. Smothers (1987/1986) examined the relationship between specific program policies, program climate as measured by the Ward Atmosphere Scale (Moos, 1989), and behavior among relatively impaired psychiatric patients. These patients tended to show more responsible behavior when they were in more structured and directive programs—that is, programs that were high on expectations for functioning, did not accept problem behavior, and were low on policy choice. In contrast, patients showed more maladaptive behavior when they were in programs that had few expectations for functioning and that tended to accept problem behavior. These findings imply that high expectations for independent behavior can have a positive influence on some impaired individuals.

Linn and colleagues (1985) followed long-term psychiatric patients who were randomly assigned to community nursing homes, VA nursing care units, or VA psychiatric units. Although less expensive, the community nursing homes also tended to have poorer outcomes than did the VA facilities. Across the different types of settings, supportive physical features and services tended to aid the more impaired residents, whereas staff resources and policies that promote resident control tended to benefit more independent residents (Timko et al., 1993).

A number of facility characteristics may work together to exert an impact on residents. For example, Manning (1989) developed overall indices of the physical and social resources in Australian group homes; these two blocks of variables explained about one third of the variance in staff-rated client outcomes, implying that, when taken together, the characteristics of the homes had a substantial influence on the residents.

Individual Environmental Perceptions and Well-Being. Several researchers have examined the associations between residents' perceptions of nursing home environments and their well-being. Prior studies have found that patients who initially held more positive views of their psychiatric program have better short- and long-term treatment outcome at follow-up (Finney & Moos, 1984, 1992).

Shadish, Orwin, Silver, and Bootzin (1985) noted that nursing home residents' well-being generally was not related to their levels of symptomatology and social integration. The strongest connections were with their appraisal of the quality of the nursing home environment; nursing home residents who saw the home as more cohesive and well organized, as oriented toward independence and resident influence, as physically comfortable, and as low in conflict and self-disclosure were likely to report higher well-being (see also Clark, 1989/1988; Colling, 1989).

Former psychiatric patients living in the community appear to benefit from involvement in decisions about program operations; those who reported sharing control with the staff were more satisfied (McCarthy & Nelson, 1991). Similarly, Earls and Nelson (1988) examined the relationship between the quality of community housing and psychological well-being among long-term psychiatric clients. More negative affect was reported by clients who experienced more concerns about their housing (as shown by an adaptation of the MEAP Rating Scale) and who had a small social network. Larger network size and positive affect were related among clients with many concerns about their housing but not among clients with few concerns. These findings show how the MEAP can be used to examine the idea of stress buffering; in this instance, the size of the social network made more difference among clients who experienced more housing-related stressors.

In a study of three homes for older adults, Orchowsky (1982) focused on the congruence between residents' actual and preferred social climates and found that residents who showed more agreement between their preferences and perceptions of the facility in the areas of conflict, self-disclosure, organization, and physical comfort reported more life satisfaction.

Similarly, Kodama (1988a, 1988b) used a Japanese version of the PAF and found that residents' complaints about physical features were predictably related to the actual physical features in their facilities. That is, the fewer the physical amenities, social-recreational aids, and so on, the higher the number of complaints in these specific areas. As expected, residents who had more complaints experienced more distress and lower morale. There also were some congruence effects. Residents who were in poorer health and who were more functionally impaired were more likely to focus on the lack of physical amenities, prosthetic aids, safety features, and space. In contrast, more active residents were more likely to focus on the lack of social-recreational aids and community accessibility.

Because these studies focused on individual residents, the relationships identified may reflect processes operating within the individual. For example, the findings may reflect a tendency for optimistic or resilient individuals, with the potential for better adjustment, to see their facility in a more positive light. Residents with a more positive outlook may elicit more support from other residents and staff and participate more actively in facility programs; as a consequence, they may develop more positive views of the social climate and experience more favorable outcomes. Whatever their source, program perceptions may provide important predictive information about individuals' later morale and well-being.

Conclusions. The preceding studies imply that group residential programs can offer a positive setting for some older individuals. Most generally, residents who are in cohesive and well-organized facilities that are oriented toward independence tend to show higher morale and well-being and to participate in more self-initiated activities in the facility and the community. A moderate level of organization and structure is also related to well-being and maintenance of functional ability.

These findings are consistent with conclusions about the effects of community-based and hospital-based psychiatric programs (Moos, 1988b, 1989). Therapeutic environments tend to be moderately supportive, to emphasize independence and personal control in an orderly and well-structured setting, and to play down the open expression of anger and aggression. Consistent with a person-environment congruence perspective, residents who are functioning marginally need a more supportive and structured setting, whereas residents who have relatively intact functioning are more sensitive to the benefits from a program that emphasizes independence and individual choice (Moos & Lemke, 1994).

FUTURE DIRECTIONS

We hold that better concepts and measures of environmental factors are needed to understand how residential settings influence health and adaptation. Supportive residential settings provide a context in which both group and individual processes operate to affect resident adaptation. Residents in a congregate living situation are part of a social entity; they share common experiences and are exposed to common environmental factors. At the same time, individual residents perceive and respond differently to the environmental features of their setting. Different processes operate at the group and individual levels; both levels should be incorporated into conceptualization and analyses.

By helping to identify the general processes by which contextual factors affect individuals, environmental assessment procedures such as the MEAP can broaden our understanding of how group residential facilities influence the individuals who live in them. These procedures can help program evaluators and managers conduct formative evaluations of residential programs, monitor stability and change, evaluate the impact of program factors, and improve programs.

Appendix A:—RESIF
Data Collection Forms

RESIDENT AND STAFF
INFORMATION FORM (RESIF)

The RESIF is one part of the Multiphasic Environmental Assessment Procedure (MEAP) for evaluating the physical and social environments of group residential facilities. It should be used with the information in Chapter 3, which provides an overview of the RESIF, instructions for organizing data collection, and item definitions. The scoring key and descriptions of the dimensions assessed by the RESIF are provided in Appendix B.

The following questions ask about (a) residents' background characteristics, (b) residents' functional abilities, (c) the type of activities in which residents participate, and (d) characteristics of the staff. Check the spaces and fill in the information requested about the facility. The word *residents* is used throughout the form; it refers to those who live in the facility (with the exception of live-in staff). Please answer the questions as fully as possible, making additional comments as necessary.

Please fill in the information below

Date _____

Name of facility _____

Type of facility (e.g., nursing home, domiciliary, residential care facility, or senior citizens apartments)

_____

How long has this facility been in operation? _____

Sponsoring agency or name of corporation _____

Your name _____

Section I:
Residents' Background Characteristics

1-3   1. How many residents are living here at present? _____

2. How many of the residents are

4-9   _____Male   _____Female

3. How many of the residents are

     _____less than 55   _____75 to 84

     _____55 to 64   _____85 and over

10-24   _____65 to 74

4. How many of the residents are

     _____Asian American   _____White

     _____Black   _____Other

25-39   _____Hispanic

5. How many of the residents come from the following religious backgrounds?

     _____Catholic   _____Other

     _____Jewish   _____None

40-54   _____Protestant

6. How many of the residents are

     _____married   _____separated or divorced

55-66   _____widowed   _____single

7. How many of the residents come from the following educational backgrounds?

     _____8th grade or less   _____Some college

     _____9th grade-12th grade   _____College graduate

1-18   _____Some post-high   _____Graduate or professional
              school education   degree

8. How many of the residents come from the following occupational backgrounds?

     _____Unskilled laborer   _____Semiprofessional

     _____Blue-collar worker   _____Manager or
              (skilled and semiskilled)   managerial worker

     _____Clerical or sales worker   _____Professional or executive

19-39   _____Homemaker or housewife

40-42   9. How many residents were not born in
            the United States? .... _____

43-45   10. How many of the residents do not speak English
            well enough to make themselves easily understood? _____

         11. For those residents who are fluent in a language other than
            English, what other languages do they speak?

            Language   Number of Residents

46-49   _____   _____

50-53   _____   _____

54-57   _____   _____

58-61   _____   _____

62-65   _____   _____

         12. If this facility is an intermediate care or skilled nursing
            facility, please answer the following questions:

1-3   12a. How many residents pay all or a portion of
                their fees with Medicare? .... _____

4-6   12b. How many residents pay all or a portion of
                their fees with Medicaid? .... _____

         13. If this facility is an apartment house or other
            sheltered living facility, please answer the
            following questions:

7-9   13a. How many residents receive
                federal rent assistance? .... _____

10-12   13b. How many residents receive Supplemental
                Security Income (SSI)? .... _____

13-15   14. How many residents receive other forms of aid? .... _____

16   Please specify type of aid: _____

         15. Indicate the number of present residents who have been
            living in the facility

            _____Less than 1 month   _____7 to 12 months

17-28   _____1 to 6 months   _____More than 12 months

29-31   16. About what proportion of prospective residents visit
            the facility before actually entering? (Do not count
            visits by residents' families.) .... _____

32-34   17. How many residents have died in the past 3 months?_____

35-37   18. How many residents have left the facility in the
             past 3 months (not counting deaths)? . . . . _____

             18a. How many of these residents went to

             _____Own home or home of   _____Nursing home
                  friends or relatives

             _____Senior citizens   _____Hospital
                  apartments

             _____Boarding home,   _____Other (please specify)
                  residential care   _____

Section II: Residents' Functional Abilities

Part I: Activities of Daily Living

	Number who do this without help	Number who do this with some help	Number unable to do this

How many residents

1-6	1. take care of their own appearance (e.g., comb hair or shave)?	_____	_____	_____
7-12	2. eat their meals?	_____	_____	_____
13-18	3. dress or undress themselves?	_____	_____	_____
19-24	4. walk?	_____	_____	_____
25-30	5. get in and out of bed?	_____	_____	_____
31-36	6. take a bath or shower?	_____	_____	_____
37-42	7. get to the bathroom on time?	_____	_____	_____
43-48	8. make their needs or wishes clearly understood?	_____	_____	_____
49-54	9. handle their own money (i.e., pay their own bills)?	_____	_____	_____
55-60	10. use the telephone?	_____	_____	_____
61-66	11. go shopping for groceries and clothes?	_____	_____	_____

Part II: Resident Disability

How many residents

1. are presently on a prescribed medication? _____ 1-3
2. do not see well enough to read a (normal print) book or newspaper (even with glasses)? _____
3. use a hearing aid or should use a hearing aid? _____
4. do not know what day and year it is? _____ 10-12

Part III: Resident Activity

During the past week, about how many residents have actually taken part in the following activities?

1. Watched TV? _____ 13-15
2. Listened to music (e.g., radio or records)? _____
3. Read a newspaper or book? _____
4. Wrote (e.g., letters, poems, etc.)? _____ 22-24
5. Sewed or knitted? _____
6. Played cards, checkers, chess, or a similar game (with others)? _____
7. Played pool, bingo, or dominoes? _____ 31-33
8. Drew or painted? _____
9. Engaged in photography, woodworking, ceramics, or other hobby? _____
10. Took care of plants or gardened? _____ 40-42
11. Visited with other residents? _____
12. Went outside on a nice day? _____
13. Took a walk? _____ 49-51

Section III: Participation in
Activities Outside the Facility

Do the residents leave the facility for any of the following activities? For each activity, indicate about how many people participate in it and how often.

		Very rarely or never 1	Only a few times a year 2	Once or twice a month 3	Once a week or more 4
1-4	1. To visit friends or relatives.....	_____	_____	_____	_____
	2. To go on a ride or tour	_____	_____	_____	_____
	3. To go to a ball game or other sports event	_____	_____	_____	_____
	4. To go on a picnic	_____	_____	_____	_____
17-20	5. To attend religious services.....	_____	_____	_____	_____
	6. To attend a funeral or memorial service	_____	_____	_____	_____
	7. To go shopping	_____	_____	_____	_____
	8. To eat in a restaurant	_____	_____	_____	_____
	9. To attend a concert or play	_____	_____	_____	_____
37-40	10. To attend the movies	_____	_____	_____	_____
	11. To go to parties	_____	_____	_____	_____
	12. To engage in volunteer or paid work.................	_____	_____	_____	_____
	13. To go on an overnight trip.....	_____	_____	_____	_____
53-56	14. To go to a senior citizens center	_____	_____	_____	_____

Section IV: Characteristics
of Staff and Volunteers

Part I: Staff

How many staff in each position are there who are hired and paid by the facility? Please answer in terms of full-time equivalents (FTEs: 40 hours per week = 1 FTE).

          1. Staff involved mainly with direct service to residents

1-4   _____ a. Registered nurses (RNs; include head nurses)

5-8   _____ b. Vocational or practical nurses

9-12   _____ c. Nurse's aides or attendants

13-15   _____ d. Physicians

16-18   _____ e. Psychologists or psychiatrists

19-21   _____ f. Social workers or other personal counselors

           _____ g. Occupational or physical therapists

25-27   _____ h. Activity directors or recreational therapists

           _____ i. Clergymen or religious counselors

31-33   _____ j. Others (please specify)_____

          2. Staff involved mainly in administrative or maintenance activities

34-36   _____ a. Administrators and supervisors

           _____ b. Office assistants or secretaries

           _____ c. Janitorial and maintenance workers

43-45   _____ d. Nutritionists, home economists, or dietitians

           _____ e. Cooks and kitchen helpers

           _____ f. Maids and room-cleaning help, or laundry workers

52-54   _____ g. Others (please specify)_____

          3. About how many of the present staff have worked in the facility

1-9   ____less than 6 months   ____6 to 12 months   ____more than
                                                  12 months

4. How many of the present staff members are

_____male 18-30   _____female 18-30

_____male 31-40   _____female 31-40

_____male 41-50   _____female 41-50

10-33   _____male 51 and over   _____female 51 and over

34   5. Do some staff who give direct services to
           residents fluently speak languages other   1   2
           than English? ....☐ Yes ☐ No

           5a. If so, please list the languages they speak
                and the number of staff who fluently speak each.

                        Language   Number who
                                                         speak it

35-38   _____   _____

39-42   _____   _____

43-46   _____   _____

47-50   _____   _____

51-54   _____   _____

                                                         1   2
55   6. Is there an in-service training program?.............☐ Yes ☐ No

           6a. If so, which of the following best describes this program?

               1
               ☐ Informal or on-the-job training only

               2 Training during orientation with continuing on-the-job
               ☐   training

               3
               ☐ Training at regular staff meetings on a continuing basis

56   4 Training at regularly scheduled meetings with programs of
               ☐ films, outside speakers, and so on.

Part II: *Volunteers*

These questions concern volunteers and the services they perform. ₁   ₂

57   1. Are there volunteers who help out in the facility?   ☐ Yes ☐ No

58-60   1a. If so, about how many different people
                 volunteer their time in a typical week?........ _____

          2. Please estimate the number of volunteer hours per week spent in

61-63   2a. activities, treatment, or other direct
                 contact with residents................................. _____

64-66   2b. other (such as administration, maintenance)_____

                                                1   2

67   3. Is there a program of training for volunteers?   ☐ Yes ☐ No

          3a. Which of the following best describes this program?

          1
          ☐ Informal or on-the-job training only

          2 Orientation for new volunteers with continuing supervision
          ☐ and on-the-job training

          3
          ☐ Ongoing, regular meetings and continuing supervision

68   4 Regularly scheduled meetings with special programs
          ☐ (e.g., outside speakers or films)

PHYSICAL AND ARCHITECTURAL
FEATURES CHECKLIST (PAF)

The PAF is one part of the Multiphasic Environmental Assessment Procedure (MEAP) for evaluating the physical and social environments of group residential facilities. It should be used with the information in Chapter 4, which provides an overview of the PAF, instructions for organizing data collection, and item definitions. The scoring key and descriptions of the dimensions assessed by the PAF are provided in Appendix B.

The following questions relate to physical characteristics inside and outside the facility and to the neighborhood context in which the facility is located. Please check the spaces and fill in the information requested about the facility. Answer the questions as fully as possible, making additional comments as necessary.

Please fill in the information below

Date _____

Name of facility _____

Type of facility (e.g., nursing home, domiciliary, residential care facility, or senior citizens apartments) _____

How long has this facility been in operation? _____

Sponsoring agency or name of corporation _____

Your name _____

This section relates to the exterior of the building and its neighborhood. Fill in the blanks or check "yes" or "no" where appropriate. There is space for additional comments at the end of each section.

Section I: Neighborhood Context

1. Is the neighborhood primarily

   1 ☐ urban

   2 ☐ suburban

   3 ☐ rural   1

       1a. If rural, how far is it to the nearest town?........ _____   2, 3

2. What type of neighborhood is the facility in?

   1 ☐ One family or low-rise apartment residential

   2 ☐ High-rise apartment residential

   3 ☐ Business

   4 ☐ Both business and residential

   5 ☐ Other (please specify) _____   4

                                                                 1   2

3. Is the facility all in one building?.................................☐ Yes ☐ No   5

   3a. If so, how many stories does the
         building have? .... _____   6, 7

   3b. How old is the building? .... _____   8, 9

4. If the facility has more than one building:

   4a. How many stories does the lowest
         building have? .... _____   10, 11

   4b. How many stories does the tallest
         building have? .... _____   12, 13

   4c. How old is the oldest of these buildings? .... _____   14, 15

5. Are the following community resources located within easy
   walking distance of the facility (1/4 mile)?

		1	2	
5a.	Grocery store	☐ Yes	☐ No	16
5b.	Drugstore	☐ Yes	☐ No	
5c.	Senior citizens center	☐ Yes	☐ No	
5d.	Movie theater	☐ Yes	☐ No	
5e.	Church or synagogue	☐ Yes	☐ No	20
5f.	Public library	☐ Yes	☐ No	
5g.	Bank	☐ Yes	☐ No	
5h.	Hospital	☐ Yes	☐ No	
5i.	Doctor's office	☐ Yes	☐ No	
5j.	Dentist's office	☐ Yes	☐ No	25
5k.	Post office	☐ Yes	☐ No	
5l.	Park	☐ Yes	☐ No	

6. Does the city or town within which this facility is
   located have a public transportation system? .... ☐ Yes ☐ No

7. Is there a public transportation stop
   within easy walking distance (1/4 mile)? .... ☐ Yes ☐ No

   7a. If so, does it have benches? .... ☐ Yes ☐ No

8. Are there lights in the surrounding streets? .... ☐ Yes ☐ No   31

Comments on the Neighborhood Context:

Items are considered applicable to all facilities except where not applicable (n.a.) is given as a possible response. Refer to the directions in the manual for the rationale and handling of specific items.

Section II: Exterior of Building

                      1   2

1. Is the main entrance sheltered from sun and rain? .... ☐ Yes ☐ No 32

2. Is the outside building area well lighted? .... ☐ Yes ☐ No

3. Are the outside walk and entrance visible

    3a. from seating spaces in the lobby or a
        ground floor social space? .... ☐ Yes ☐ No

    3b. from the office or station of an employee? .... ☐ Yes ☐ No 35

4. Is there outside seating in the front
   of the building? .... ☐ Yes ☐ No

    4a. Is it visible from the entrance lobby or a
        ground floor social space? .... ☐ n.a. ☐ Yes ☐ No

    4b. Is it visible from the office or station of
        an employee? .... ☐ n.a. ☐ Yes ☐ No

    4c. Is it protected from the weather? .... ☐ Yes ☐ No

    4d. Does it provide a view of pedestrians and
        other activity? .... ☐ Yes ☐ No 40

5. Is there a patio or open courtyard? .... ☐ Yes ☐ No

6. If there is an outside area:

    6a. Are tables available? .... ☐ Yes ☐ No

    6b. Are umbrella tables available? .... ☐ Yes ☐ No

    6c. Is the outdoor furniture in good condition? .... ☐ Yes ☐ No

    6d. Is there a covered area (rainproof)? .... ☐ Yes ☐ No 45

    6e. Is there an area with a sun screen
        (not necessarily rainproof) or protection
        from the sun (e.g., trees)? .... ☐ Yes ☐ No

    6f. Is there a barbecue? .... ☐ Yes ☐ No

    6g. Is there a shuffleboard game area? .... ☐ Yes ☐ No 48

  7. Is there a garden area for resident use? ....☐ Yes ☐ No 49

  8. Is there a lawn?...☐ Yes ☐ No 50

  9. Is there parking reserved for handicapped?.................☐ Yes ☐ No

10. Is there parking for staff? ....☐ Yes ☐ No

11. Is there parking for visitors?...☐ Yes ☐ No 53

12. What is the acreage of the grounds?............................ _____ 54-57

Comments on the Exterior of the Building:

Section III: Interior of Building

Part I: Lobby and Entrance Area

1. Can one enter the building from the street
   without having to use any stairs?..................☐ Yes   ☐ No 1

2. Is the entry from outside limited to one
   unlocked door?..................☐ Yes   ☐ No

3. Is there a bell or call system outside?..................☐ Yes   ☐ No

4. Are written instructions posted outside that explain
   how to get in if the front door is locked?..................☐ Yes   ☐ No

5. Does the front door open automatically?..................☐ Yes   ☐ No 5

6. Does the front door swing closed by itself?..................☐ Yes   ☐ No

7. Is the front door wide enough for a wheelchair?..................☐ Yes   ☐ No

8. Is there an individual who usually monitors access
   to the building?..................☐ Yes   ☐ No

9. Is there a reception area or reception desk?..................☐ Yes   ☐ No

10. Is there a place for visitors to sign in?..................☐ Yes   ☐ No 10

11. Is there a lobby?..................☐ Yes   ☐ No

     11a. If so, approximately what size is it?........._____ sq. ft.   12-15

12. Is there seating in the lobby?..................☐ Yes   ☐ No 16

13. Is there a lounge near the entrance
    (other than the lobby)?..................☐ Yes   ☐ No

     13a. If so, is this lounge furnished for resting
    or casual conversation?..................☐ Yes   ☐ No

14. Can one see into the lobby or entrance area from a
    lounge or other ground floor social space?..................☐ Yes   ☐ No

15. Is there a large face clock in the lobby or
    entrance area?..................☐ Yes   ☐ No 20

Comments on the Interior of the Building:

Part II: Hall and Stairway Areas

1. How wide are the hallways (in feet)? .... _____   21

2. Are the hallways crowded or are there
   obstructions (e.g., wheelchairs, meal carts,   1   2
   or cleaning equipment)? ....☐ Yes   ☐ No

3. Are there handrails in the halls? ....☐ Yes   ☐ No

4. Are the halls decorated (e.g., pictures or plants)?..........☐ Yes   ☐ No

5. Are there drinking fountains?...☐ Yes   ☐ No 25

   5a. If so, how many per floor? ...._____

   5b. Are they accessible to wheelchair residents?...........☐ Yes   ☐ No

6. Are there public telephones? ....☐ Yes   ☐ No

   6a. If so, how many per floor? ...._____

   6b. Is there a writing surface by the telephone? ....☐ Yes   ☐ No 30

   6c. Is at least one telephone accessible to
       wheelchair residents?...☐ Yes   ☐ No

   6d. Does at least one telephone have a loudness
       control in the receiver for people who are
       hard of hearing? ....☐ Yes   ☐ No

7. Are there smoke detection devices in the halls?.............☐ Yes   ☐ No

8. Does a resident have to climb any steps to have
   access to all areas of the building intended for
   resident use? ....☐ Yes   ☐ No

                                                     0
9. Are the stairs well lighted? ....☐ n. a. ☐ Yes   ☐ No 35

10. Are there nonskid surfaces on stairs and ramps?..☐ n. a. ☐ Yes   ☐ No

11. Is each floor or corridor color coded or numbered? .....☐ Yes   ☐ No

12. Are the residents' names on or next to their doors?......☐ Yes   ☐ No

13. Is it relatively easy for new residents to find their
    way around the building—that is, is the building
    well marked or small and uncomplicated? ....☐ Yes   ☐ No 39

Comments on the Hall and Stairway Areas:

Parts III, IV, and V cover the communal rooms in the facility. Three categories are used: lounge or community room areas, recreational or special activity areas, and dining room areas. Each room should be listed under only one category according to its main function.

Part III: Lounge and Community Room Areas

	1	2	
1. Are there any lounge or community room areas?..........	☐ Yes	☐ No	40
1a. If so, how many? ...._____			41-43
1b. What size is the smallest lounge?.............._____ sq. ft.			44-47
1c. What size is the largest lounge? ...._____ sq. ft.			48-51
1d. How large are the lounges all together?...._____ sq. ft.			52-55
2. Are any of these rooms near an entrance or traveled hallway?	☐ Yes	☐ No	56
3. Are there writing desks or tables?..................	☐ Yes	☐ No	
4. Are there small tables for several people to sit and talk or play games?	☐ Yes	☐ No	
5. Is reading material available on tables or shelves?.........	☐ Yes	☐ No	
6. Are there any table lamps?..............................	☐ Yes	☐ No	60
7. Is the furniture spaced wide enough for wheelchairs?...	☐ Yes	☐ No	
8. Is there a quiet lounge with no television?	☐ Yes	☐ No	62

Comments on the Lounge and Community Room Areas:

Part IV: Recreation or Special Activity Areas

1. Are there any areas primarily designated for
   recreation or special activities? (Do not record these
   areas under any other category.) .... ☐ Yes ☐ No 1

   1a. If so, how many? ...._____ 2-4

   1b. What size is the smallest such area? ...._____sq. ft. 5-8

   1c. What size is the largest such area? ...._____sq. ft. 9-12

   1d. How large are these areas all together?....._____sq. ft. 13-16

2. Is there a library from which books can
   be borrowed? .... ☐ Yes ☐ No 17

3. Is there a music or listening room?.............................. ☐ Yes ☐ No

   What types of recreational or special activity materials are available?

4. Pool or billiard table? .... ☐ Yes ☐ No

5. Ping-pong table? .... ☐ Yes ☐ No 20

6. Piano or organ? .... ☐ Yes ☐ No

7. One or more television sets?.. ☐ Yes ☐ No

8. One or more phonographs?... ☐ Yes ☐ No

9. One or more radios?.. ☐ Yes ☐ No

10. One or more sewing machines?...................................... ☐ Yes ☐ No 25

Comments on Recreation or Special Activity Areas:

Part V: Dining Room Areas

1. Are there any dining areas? .... ☐ Yes ☐ No 26

   1a. If so, how many? (Do not record these areas
       under any other category.) ...._____ 27-29

   1b. What size is the smallest dining room?......_____sq. ft. 30-33

   1c. What size is the largest dining room?........_____sq. ft. 34-37

   1d. How large are these areas all together? ......_____sq. ft. 38-41

2. Are there small tables that seat fewer than six? ....☐ Yes ☐ No 42

3. Are there large tables that seat more than six? ....☐ Yes ☐ No

4. Is aisle space between tables at least 60 inches?............☐ Yes ☐ No

Comments on Dining Room Areas:

Part VI: Staff and Office Areas

1. Are there offices for the administrative staff?................☐ Yes ☐ No 45

2. Is there office space for the secretarial and
   clerical staff?..☐ Yes ☐ No

3. Are there offices for social service and
   counseling staff? ....☐ Yes ☐ No

4. Is there additional office space available for
   other staff (e.g., activity director, volunteers,
   or part-time staff)? ....☐ Yes ☐ No

5. Are the offices free of distractions from
   adjacent activities?...☐ Yes ☐ No

6. Is there a separate room for handling mail,
   copying, or printing? ....☐ Yes ☐ No 50

7. Is there a conference room? ....☐ Yes ☐ No

8. Is there a staff lounge?..☐ Yes ☐ No

   8a. If so, does it have tables? ....☐ Yes ☐ No

   8b. Does it have comfortable chairs?...........................☐ Yes ☐ No

   8c. What size is it?.._____ sq. ft.   55-58

9. How many staff members are there all together
   (in FTEs: 1 FTE = 40 hours/week)? .... _____   59-61

Comments on Staff and Office Areas:

Part VII: General Facilities

1. Is a map showing community resources available
   in a convenient public location? ....☐ Yes ☐ No 1

2. Is there a bulletin board in a public location?................☐ Yes ☐ No

3. Is there a posted list of the staff? ....☐ Yes ☐ No

   3a. If so, does it include pictures? ....☐ Yes ☐ No

4. Is there a posted list of residents?.................................☐ Yes ☐ No 5

   4a. If so, does it include pictures? ....☐ Yes ☐ No

5. Is there a sound system or public address system?.........☐ Yes ☐ No

6. Is there an air-conditioning system? ....☐ Yes ☐ No

7. Is there a chapel or meditation room?...........................☐ Yes ☐ No

8. Is there a gift shop, commissary, or store? ....☐ Yes ☐ No10

9. Is there a kitchen area in which a resident or
   visitor can make a cup of coffee, heat some
   soup, or the like?...☐ Yes ☐ No

10. Is there a snack bar? ....☐ Yes ☐ No

11. Are there vending machines for
    candy or soft drinks? ....☐ Yes ☐ No

    11a. If so, are they used by residents? ....☐ Yes ☐ No

12. Is there a laundry area for residents' use?......................☐ Yes ☐ No 15

Comments on General Facilities:

Part VIII: Bathroom and Toilet Areas

	All or almost all	Some	Very few or none	
	1	2	3	
1. Are there raised thresholds at the entrances?	☐	☐	☐	
2. Do the bathroom doors open out?	☐	☐	☐	16
3. Are there handrails or safety bars?	☐	☐	☐	
4. Are there lift bars next to the toilet?	☐	☐	☐	
5. Are the towel racks and dispensers higher than 40 inches from the floor?	☐	☐	☐	
6. Are there mirrors in the bathrooms?	☐	☐	☐	20
7. Are there nonslip surfaces in all areas subject to wetness?	☐	☐	☐	
8. Are there call buttons in the bathrooms?	☐	☐	☐	
9. Is there turning radius for a wheelchair (5 feet × 5 feet)?	☐	☐	☐	

10. What size is the smallest bathroom? _____sq. ft. 25-27

11. What size is the largest bathroom? _____sq. ft. 28-30

12. What is the largest number of residents who share one bathroom area? _____ 31, 32

13. Does each resident have access to both a bathtub and a shower? ☐ Yes ☐ No 33

    13a. How many bathtubs are there? . . . . _____ 34-36

    13b. How many showers are there? . . . . _____ 37-39

    13c. Is there a flexible shower? . . . . ☐ Yes ☐ No 40

    13d. Is there a seat included in the shower? . . . . ☐ Yes ☐ No 41

    13e. Is a wheelchair-entered shower available? . . ☐ Yes ☐ No 42

Comments on the Bathroom and Toilet Areas:

Part IX: Individual Rooms or Apartments

1. How many rooms or apartments or both are
   there all together? .... _____   1-3

2. How many residents are living here at the
   present time? .... _____   4-6

3. What is the largest number of residents who
   share one room or apartment? .... _____   7, 8

Are the following features present in individual rooms or apartments?

	All or almost all	Some	Very few or none
	1	2	3
4. Is there wall space available on which residents can hang pictures?	☐	☐	☐ 9
5. Are there wall lights (or table lamps) that give adequate light for reading?	☐	☐	☐ 10
6. Is there a mirror?	☐	☐	☐
7. Is there a window sill that is wide enough for flowers?	☐	☐	☐
8. Are the floors a light color?	☐	☐	☐
9. Are the walls a light color?	☐	☐	☐
10. Are there individual heating controls?	☐	☐	☐ 15
11. Are there individual air-conditioning controls?	☐	☐	☐
12. Is there a telephone or a telephone connection?	☐	☐	☐
13. Is there room for wheelchair use?	☐	☐	☐
14. Are there handrails?	☐	☐	☐
15. Are there smoke detection devices?	☐	☐	☐ 20
16. Is there a call button or telephone connection in every room (e.g., each bedroom of two-bedroom apartments)?	☐	☐	☐

	All or almost all	*Some*	*Very few or none*

N/A

17. Do the apartments have their
    own kitchen or kitchenette? . . . . □   □   □   □ 22

    (0)

18. What size is the smallest room or apartment? .... _____ sq. ft. 23-26

19. What size is the largest room or apartment? .... _____ sq. ft. 27-30

20. What size is the smallest per person closet area? ... _____ sq. ft. 31-32

21. What size is the largest per person closet area? ..... _____ sq. ft. 33-34

Comments on Individual Rooms or Apartments:

POLICY AND PROGRAM
INFORMATION FORM (POLIF)

The POLIF is one part of the Multiphasic Environmental Assessment Procedure (MEAP) for evaluating the physical and social environments of group residential facilities. It should be used with the information in Chapter 5, which provides an overview of the POLIF, instructions for organizing data collection, and item definitions. The scoring key and descriptions of the dimensions assessed by the POLIF are provided in Appendix B.

The following questions ask about (a) the financial and entrance arrangements, (b) the types of rooms or apartments in the facility, (c) the way in which the facility is organized, and (d) the services provided for residents. Please check the boxes and fill in the information requested. The word *residents* is used throughout the form; it refers to those who live in the facility (with the exception of live-in staff). Please answer the questions as fully as possible, making additional comments as necessary.

Please fill in the information below

Date _____

Name of facility _____

Type of facility (e.g., nursing home, domiciliary, residential care facility, or senior citizens apartments) _____

How long has this facility been in operation? _____

Sponsoring agency or name of corporation _____

Your name _____

Section I: Financial and Entrance Arrangements

	1	2

1. Is there an initial entrance fee? ....□ Yes   □ No   1

    1a. If so, what is the minimum fee?

       1 □ Less than $1,000

       2 □ $1,000 to $4,999

       3 □ $5,000 to $9,999

       4 □ $10,000 or more   2

2. What is the minimum monthly rate for residents who are not receiving federal or state aid?

       1 □ Less than $200

       2 □ $200 to $399

       3 □ $400 to $599

       4 □ $600 to $799

       5 □ $800 or more   3

    2a. What services are covered by this monthly rate?

       □ Room   □ Cleaning or   □ Personal care   4-8

                             maid service

       □ Board   □ Nursing care

3. Are rates set on a sliding scale based on the   1   2   9
resident's income? ....□ Yes   □ No

4. Must a prospective resident be ambulatory? ....□ Yes   □ No 10

5. Is there a minimum age requirement? ....□ Yes   □ No

    5a. If so, what is it? .... _____   12,13

6. Is there a waiting list for this facility?...........................□ Yes   □ No 14

    6a. If so, about how many people are on it? .... _____   15-17

7. What is the total capacity of the facility—i.e., how many residents can live here all together)?.................... _____   18-20

8. How many residents are living in the facility at the present time? .... _____   21-23

Section II: Types of Rooms and Features Available

1. If this facility is divided into rooms or dormitories,
   please answer the following questions:

   1a. What is the total number of rooms for residents? .. _____ 24-26

   1b. How many private rooms are there? .... _____

   1c. How many rooms are there with two residents? .... _____

   1d. How many rooms are there with three residents? .. _____ 33-35

   1e. How many rooms are there with four or more
        residents? .... _____

   1f. What is the largest number of residents who
        share one room or dormitory unit? .... _____

   1g. How many private bathrooms are there? .... _____ 42-44

   1h. How many bathrooms are shared by two residents? _____

   1i. How many bathrooms are shared by three
        or more residents? .... _____

   1j. What is the largest number of residents who
        share one bathroom area? .... _____ 51-53

2. If this facility is divided into apartments:

   2a. How many apartments are there for residents? ...... _____

   2b. How many studio apartments are there? .... _____

   2c. How many one-bedroom apartments are there? .... _____ 60-62

   2d. How many two-bedroom apartments are there? .... _____

3. For all facilities: 1   2

   3a. Are there furnished rooms or apartments? .... ☐ Yes   ☐ No 66

   3b. Do residents have their own individual
        mailboxes? .... ☐ Yes   ☐ No

   3c. Is there a dresser for each person? .... ☐ Yes   ☐ No

   3d. Are there locks on all bathroom doors? .... ☐ Yes   ☐ No 69

Section III: Organizational Policies

Part I: General Information

1. Which of the following best describes the ownership
   and management of the facility?

    1 ☐ Individual or partnership

    2 ☐ Nonprofit organization

    3 ☐ Government or public

    4 ☐ Large corporation

    5 ☐ Small corporation

    6 ☐ Management company

    7 ☐ Other (please specify) _____   1

                                                       1   2

2. Does this facility have a board of directors?................. ☐ Yes   ☐ No 2

    2a. If so, how many members are on the board?.......... _____ 3-4

    2b. How often does the board meet?

    1 ☐ Once a month or more

    2 ☐ Quarterly or bimonthly

    3 ☐ Once or twice a year or less   5

3. If there is a board of directors, does it have
   a say in any of the approaches used or the
   activities provided in the facility? .... ☐ Yes   ☐ No 6

4. Do some of the staff, other than the administrator,
   regularly attend board meetings? .... ☐ Yes   ☐ No

5. Is there a handbook for residents
   (e.g., rules, medical procedures, etc.)?........................... ☐ Yes   ☐ No

6. Is there a handbook for staff (e.g., policies, operating
   procedures, and treatment approaches)?....................... ☐ Yes   ☐ No

7. Does the facility have an orientation program
   for new residents? .... ☐ Yes   ☐ No

8. Is there an orientation program for new staff?.............. ☐ Yes   ☐ No 11

9. Are there formal staff meetings?....................☐¹ Yes   ☐² No 12

    9a. If so, how often?

        1 ☐ Once a week or more

        2 ☐ Once or twice a month

        3 ☐ Less than once a month

        4 ☐ Only when needed   13

10. Are there volunteers who help out in the facility?.........☐ Yes   ☐ No

    10a. If so, is there an orientation program   0
        for volunteers? ....☐ n.a. ☐ Yes   ☐ No 15

Part II: Rules Related to
Personal Possessions and Behaviors

This section includes questions about the rules and expectations for residents. Check the boxes that best describe the policies and procedures in this facility. The following categories are used for Part II.

1. Encouraged   —this kind of behavior or activity is encouraged here.
2. Allowed   —this kind of behavior is expected; no special attempt is made to change it.
3. Discouraged   —an attempt is made to discourage or to try to stop this behavior.
4. Intolerable   —a person who persisted in this type of behavior would probably have to move out.

	Encouraged	Allowed	Discouraged	Intolerable
	1	2	3	4
1. Drinking liquor in one's room....... ☐		☐	☐	☐ 16
2. Having one's own furniture in the room.................................. ☐		☐	☐	☐
3. Moving furniture around the room...................................... ☐		☐	☐	☐
4. Keeping a fish or bird in the room ☐		☐	☐	☐
5. Keeping a hot plate or coffee maker in the room......................... ☐		☐	☐	☐ 20
6. Doing some laundry in the bathroom (e.g., washing socks or underwear)............................... ☐		☐	☐	☐
7. Drinking a glass of wine or beer at meals..................................... ☐		☐	☐	☐
8. Skipping breakfast to sleep late...... ☐		☐	☐	☐
9. Closing the door to one's room..... ☐		☐	☐	☐
10. Locking the door to one's room ...... ☐		☐	☐	☐ 25

For Parts III and IV, please use the following categories to describe the facility's policies with respect to these behaviors and activities:

1. Allowed—   this kind of behavior is expected; no special attempt is made to change it.

2. Tolerated—   this kind of behavior is expected, but an effort is made to encourage the individual to function better or more appropriately.

3. Discouraged—   an attempt is made to discourage or to try to stop this behavior.

4. Intolerable—   a person who persisted in this type of behavior would probably have to move out.

Part III: Expectations Relating to Level of Functional Ability

	Allowed	Tolerated	Discouraged	Intolerable
	1	2	3	4
1. Inability to make one's own bed	☐	☐	☐	☐ 26
2. Inability to clean one's own room	☐	☐	☐	☐
3. Inability to feed oneself	☐	☐	☐	☐
4. Inability to bathe or clean oneself	☐	☐	☐	☐
5. Inability to dress oneself	☐	☐	☐	☐ 30
6. Incontinence (of urine or feces)	☐	☐	☐	☐
7. Confusion or disorientation	☐	☐	☐	☐
8. Depression (i.e., frequent crying or sadness)	☐	☐	☐	☐ 33

Part IV: Rules Related to
Potential "Problem" Behaviors

	Allowed	Tolerated	Discouraged	Intolerable
	1	2	3	4
1. Refusing to participate in programmed activities	☐	☐	☐	☐ 1
2. Refusing to take prescribed medicine	☐	☐	☐	☐
3. Taking medicine other than that which is prescribed	☐	☐	☐	☐
4. Taking too much medicine, intentionally or otherwise	☐	☐	☐	☐
5. Being drunk	☐	☐	☐	☐ 5
6. Wandering around the building or grounds at night	☐	☐	☐	☐
7. Leaving the building during the evening without letting anyone know	☐	☐	☐	☐
8. Refusing to bathe or clean oneself regularly	☐	☐	☐	☐
9. Creating a disturbance; being noisy or boisterous	☐	☐	☐	☐
10. Pilfering or stealing others' belongings	☐	☐	☐	☐ 10
11. Damaging or destroying property (e.g., tearing books or magazines)	☐	☐	☐	☐
12. Verbally threatening another resident	☐	☐	☐	☐
13. Physically attacking another resident	☐	☐	☐	☐
14. Physically attacking a staff member	☐	☐	☐	☐
15. Attempting suicide	☐	☐	☐	☐ 15
16. Indecently exposing self	☐	☐	☐	☐ 16

Part V: Resident Participation

1. Are any of the residents hired and paid for jobs
   within the facility?... □ Yes   □ No 17

2. Do any of the residents have other types of chores
   or duties (unpaid) that they perform here? .... □ Yes   □ No 18

   2a. If so, how many residents participate? _____   19-20

3. Is there a residents' council (i.e., residents who are
   elected or volunteer to represent residents at
   regularly scheduled meetings)?..................................... □ Yes   □ No 21

   3a. If so, how many residents are on it? ...._____   22-23

   3b. How often does it meet?

      1 □ Once a week or more

      2 □ Twice a month

      3 □ Once a month or less   24

4. Are there regular "house meetings" for residents
   (a general meeting open to all residents)? .... □ Yes   □ No 25

   4a. If so, how often do they occur?

      1 □ Twice a month or more

      2 □ Once a month

      3 □ Less than once a month

      4 □ Only when needed .... □ Yes   □ No 26

5. Are there resident committees (or committees that include residents as members)? .... ☐ Yes   ☐ No 27

   5a. If so, list the most important committees, the number of residents on each, and how often they meet.

Committee Name	Number of Residents	Frequency	
_____	_____	_____	28-31
_____	_____	_____	32-35
_____	_____	_____	36-39
_____	_____	_____	40-43
_____	_____	_____	44-47

6. Is there a newsletter? .... ☐ Yes   ☐ No 48

   6a. If so, how often is it printed?

     1 ☐ Once a week or more

     2 ☐ Twice a month

     3 ☐ Once a month

     4 ☐ Less than once a month   49

   6b. If so, is it primarily written by residents? .... ☐ Yes   ☐ No 50

7. Is there a bulletin board? .... ☐ Yes   ☐ No

   7a. If so, is it being used by residents? .... ☐ Yes   ☐ No

   7b. Are rules and regulations posted on the bulletin board or in another convenient public location? .... ☐ Yes   ☐ No 53

Part VI: Decision Making

To what extent are residents involved in policy making in the following areas?

	Staff/administration basically decide by themselves	Staff/administration decide but residents have input	Residents decide but staff has input	Residents basically decide by themselves
	1	2	3	4
1. Planning entertainment such as movies or parties	☐	☐	☐	☐54
2. Planning educational activities such as courses and lectures	☐	☐	☐	☐
3. Planning welcoming or orientation activities	☐	☐	☐	☐
4. Deciding what kinds of new activities or programs will occur	☐	☐	☐	☐
5. Making rules about attendance at activities	☐	☐	☐	☐
6. Planning daily or weekly menus	☐	☐	☐	☐
7. Setting mealtimes	☐	☐	☐	☐60
8. Setting visitors' hours	☐	☐	☐	☐
9. Deciding on the decor of public areas (e.g., pictures, plants, etc.)	☐	☐	☐	☐
10. Dealing with safety hazards	☐	☐	☐	☐
11. Dealing with residents' complaints	☐	☐	☐	☐
12. Making rules about the use of alcohol	☐	☐	☐	☐65
13. Selecting new residents	☐	☐	☐	☐
14. Moving a resident from one bed or room to another	☐	☐	☐	☐
15. Deciding when a troublesome or sick resident will be asked to leave	☐	☐	☐	☐
16. Changes in staff (hiring or firing)	☐	☐	☐	☐69

Section IV: Services and Activities Available

Part I: Services

Please indicate which of the following services are provided by this facility and the approximate number of residents who use them.

Service			Approximate number of residents who use this service at least once in a typical week	
	1	2		
1. Regularly scheduled doctor's hours	☐ Yes	☐ No	_____	1-3
2. Doctor on call	☐ Yes	☐ No	_____	
3. Regularly scheduled nurse's hours	☐ Yes	☐ No	_____	
4. Assistance in using prescribed medications	☐ Yes	☐ No	_____	10-12
5. On-site medical clinic	☐ Yes	☐ No	_____	
6. Physical therapy	☐ Yes	☐ No	_____	
7. Occupational therapy	☐ Yes	☐ No	_____	19-21
8. Psychotherapy or personal counseling	☐ Yes	☐ No	_____	
9. Religious advice or counseling	☐ Yes	☐ No	_____	
10. Legal advice or counseling	☐ Yes	☐ No	_____	28-30
11. Assistance with banking or other financial matters	☐ Yes	☐ No	_____	
12. Assistance with housekeeping or cleaning	☐ Yes	☐ No	_____	
13. Assistance with preparing meals	☐ Yes	☐ No	_____	37-39
14. Assistance with personal care or grooming	☐ Yes	☐ No	_____	
15. Barber or beauty service	☐ Yes	☐ No	_____	
16. Assistance with laundry or linen service	☐ Yes	☐ No	_____	46-48
17. Assistance with shopping	☐ Yes	☐ No	_____	
18. Providing transportation (e.g., minibus or pickup car)	☐ Yes	☐ No	_____	
19. Handling spending money for residents	☐ Yes	☐ No	_____	55-57

Part II: Additional Services and Procedures

1. Is breakfast served each day? ....☐¹Yes   ☐²No   ☐³M-F only 1

   1a. What hours is breakfast served? ...._____ 2

   1b. How many residents use this service on a typical day?_____ 3-4

2. Is lunch served each day? ....☐¹Yes   ☐²No   ☐³M-F only 5

   2a. What hours is lunch served?.._____ 6

   2b. How many residents use this service on a typical day?_____ 7-8

3. Is dinner served each day? ....☐¹Yes   ☐²No   ☐³M-F only 9

   3a. What hours is dinner served? ...._____ 10

   3b. How many residents use this service on a typical day?_____11-12

4. Are snacks served in the afternoon or evening?   ☐¹Yes   ☐²No   13

   4a. How many residents use this service on a typical day?_____14-15

5. Can residents choose to sit wherever
   they want at meals?...☐Yes   ☐No

6. Does a staff member take attendance or count
   residents at mealtimes? ....☐Yes   ☐No

7. Is there a fairly set time at which residents are
   awakened in the morning?.....................................☐Yes   ☐No   18

   7a. If so, what time?

      1☐ Before 7:00

      2☐ Between 7:00 and 8:00

      3☐ Between 8:00 and 9:00

      4☐ 9:00 or later   19

8. Are there certain times during which residents
   are expected to take baths or showers? ....☐Yes   ☐No   20

9. Is there a fairly set time at which residents
   are expected to go to bed (lights out) at night? ....☐ Yes ☐ No 21

   9a. If so, what time?

   1 ☐ Before 8:00

   2 ☐ Between 8:00 and 9:00

   3 ☐ Between 9:00 and 10:00

   4 ☐ 10:00 or later 22

10. Is there a "curfew" (i.e., a time by which all
    residents must be in the facility in the evening)? ..☐ Yes ☐ No 23

    10a. If so, what time?

    1 ☐ Before 9:00

    2 ☐ Between 9:00 and 10:00

    3 ☐ Between 10:00 and 11:00

    4 ☐ 11:00 or later 24

11. Does the staff take a count or make a check
    each day to be sure that none of the residents
    are missing? ....☐ Yes ☐ No 25

12. Are some areas of the building locked or out of
    bounds to residents at times (e.g., the dining area,
    the crafts room, certain lounges or stairways)?.....☐ Yes ☐ No 26

13. Are there regular visiting hours?...........................☐ Yes ☐ No

    13a. If so, what are the hours on a weekday? .... _____ 28

14. Are there offices that are closed and private that can
    be used for interviewing residents?.......................☐ Yes ☐ No

15. Is background music played in the building? ....☐ Yes ☐ No 30

Part III: Activities
That Take Place in the Facility

For each activity, indicate the frequency of occurrence and about how many residents participate.

	Very rarely or never	Only a few times a year	Once or twice a month	Once a week or more	About how many residents participate?
	1	2	3	4	
1. Exercises or other physical fitness activity .... ☐	☐	☐	☐		_____ 31-33
2. Outside entertainment (e.g., pianist or singer) .... ☐	☐	☐	☐		_____
3. Discussion groups .... ☐	☐	☐	☐		_____
4. Reality orientation group ..... ☐	☐	☐	☐		_____ 40-42
5. Self-help or mutual support group .... ☐	☐	☐	☐		_____
6. Films or movies .... ☐	☐	☐	☐		_____
7. Club, social group, or drama or singing groups ...... ☐	☐	☐	☐		_____ 49-51
8. Classes or lectures .... ☐	☐	☐	☐		_____
9. Bingo, cards, or other games .... ☐	☐	☐	☐		_____
10. Parties .... ☐	☐	☐	☐		_____ 58-60
11. Religious services .... ☐	☐	☐	☐		_____
12. Social hour (e.g., coffee or cocktail hour) .... ☐	☐	☐	☐		_____
13. Arts and crafts .... ☐	☐	☐	☐		_____ 67-69

SHELTERED CARE
ENVIRONMENT SCALE FORM R

Name (optional)_____ Age_____

Name of facility_____

☐ Male   ☐ Female

How long have you lived or worked here? _____ _____ _____
                                           Years   Months   Days

If you are a staff member, check the following box ☐
and indicate your staff position _____

Today's date _____

    There are 63 questions here. They are statements about the place in which you live or work. Based on your experience here, please answer these questions yes or no. Ask yourself which answer is generally true.

    Circle yes if you think the statement is true or mostly true of this place.

    Circle no if you think the statement is false or mostly false of this place.

    Please be sure to answer every question. Thank you for your cooperation.

1. Do residents get a lot of individual attention?..........................Yes   No

2. Do residents ever start arguments?...Yes   No

3. Do residents usually depend on the staff to set
   up activities for them?..Yes   No

4. Are residents careful about what they say to
   each other?...Yes   No

5. Do residents always know when the staff
   will be around?..Yes   No

6. Is the staff strict about rules and regulations? ....Yes   No

7. Is the furniture here comfortable and homey? ....Yes   No

8. Do staff members spend a lot of time with residents?.............Yes   No

9. Is it unusual for residents to openly express
   their anger? ....Yes   No

10. Do residents usually wait for staff to suggest
    an idea or activity? ....Yes   No

11. Are personal problems openly talked about?...........................Yes   No

12. Are activities for residents carefully planned? ....Yes   No

13. Are new and different ideas often tried out? ....Yes   No

14. Is it ever cold and drafty here? ....Yes   No

15. Do staff members sometimes talk down to residents? ....Yes   No

16. Do residents sometimes criticize or make fun
    of this place? ....Yes   No

17. Are residents taught how to deal with
    practical problems? ....Yes   No

18. Do residents tend to hide their feelings
    from one another?...Yes   No

19. Do some residents look messy? ....Yes   No

20. If two residents fight with each other will
    they get in trouble?...Yes   No

21. Can residents have privacy whenever they want?....................Yes   No

22. Are there a lot of social activities? ....Yes   No

23. Do residents usually keep their disagreements
    to themselves? ....Yes   No

24. Are many new skills taught here? .... Yes   No

25. Do residents talk a lot about their fears? .... Yes   No

26. Do things always seem to be changing around here? .... Yes   No

27. Do staff allow the residents to break minor rules? .... Yes   No

28. Does this place seem crowded? .... Yes   No

29. Do a lot of the residents just seem to be
    passing time here? .... Yes   No

30. Is it unusual for residents to complain about
    each other? .... Yes   No

31. Are residents learning to do more things on
    their own? .... Yes   No

32. Is it hard to tell how the residents are feeling? .... Yes   No

33. Do residents know what will happen to them if
    they break a rule? .... Yes   No

34. Are suggestions made by the residents acted on? .... Yes   No

35. Is it sometimes very noisy here? .... Yes   No

36. Are requests made by residents usually taken care
    of right away? .... Yes   No

37. Is it always peaceful and quiet here? .... Yes   No

38. Are the residents strongly encouraged to make
    their own decisions? .... Yes   No

39. Do residents talk a lot about their past dreams
    and ambitions? .... Yes   No

40. Is there a lot of confusion here at times? .... Yes   No

41. Do residents have any say in making the rules? .... Yes   No

42. Does it ever smell bad here? .... Yes   No

43. Do staff members sometimes criticize residents
    over minor things? .... Yes   No

44. Do residents often get impatient with each other? .... Yes   No

45. Do residents sometimes take charge of activities? .... Yes   No

46. Do residents ever talk about illness and death? .... Yes   No

47. Is this place very well organized? .... Yes   No

48. Are the rules and regulations rather strictly enforced? .... Yes   No

49. Is it ever hot and stuffy in here? ....Yes   No

50. Do residents tend to keep to themselves here? ....Yes   No

51. Do residents complain a lot? ....Yes   No

52. Do residents care more about the past than the future? ....Yes   No

53. Do residents talk about their money problems? ....Yes   No

54. Are things sometimes unclear around here? ....Yes   No

55. Would a resident ever be asked to leave if he or
    she broke a rule? ....Yes   No

56. Is the lighting very good here? ....Yes   No

57. Are the discussions very interesting? ....Yes   No

58. Do residents criticize each other a lot? ....Yes   No

59. Are some of the residents' activities really
    challenging? ....Yes   No

60. Do residents keep their personal problems to
    themselves? ....Yes   No

61. Are people always changing their minds around here? ....Yes   No

62. Can residents change things here if they really try? ....Yes   No

63. Do the colors and decorations make this a
    warm and cheerful place? ....Yes   No

SHELTERED CARE ENVIRONMENT SCALE—
ANSWER SHEET

Name (optional)_____ Age_____
Name of Facility_____

☐ Male   ☐ Female   Today's Date_____
How long have you lived or worked here? _____ _____ _____
                               Years   Months   Days
If you are a staff member, check the following box ☐
and indicate your staff position_____

	Item 1	Item 2	Item 3	Item 4	Item 5	Item 6	Item 7	
Yes								Yes
No								No
	Item 8	Item 9	Item 10	Item 11	Item 12	Item 13	Item 14	
Yes								Yes
No								No
	Item 15	Item 16	Item 17	Item 18	Item 19	Item 20	Item 21	
Yes								Yes
No								No
	Item 22	Item 23	Item 24	Item 25	Item 26	Item 27	Item 28	
Yes								Yes
No								No
	Item 29	Item 30	Item 31	Item 32	Item 33	Item 34	Item 35	
Yes								Yes
No								No
	Item 36	Item 37	Item 38	Item 39	Item 40	Item 41	Item 42	
Yes								Yes
No								No
	Item 43	Item 44	Item 45	Item 46	Item 47	Item 48	Item 49	
Yes								Yes
No								No
	Item 50	Item 51	Item 52	Item 53	Item 54	Item 55	Item 56	
Yes								Yes
No								No
	Item 57	Item 58	Item 59	Item 60	Item 61	Item 62	Item 63	
Yes								Yes
No								No

RATING SCALE

This Rating Scale is one part of the Multiphasic Environmental Assessment Procedure (MEAP) for evaluating the physical and social environments of group residential facilities. It should be used with the information in Chapter 7, which provides an overview of the Rating Scale, instructions for organizing data collection, and item definitions. The scoring key and descriptions of the dimensions assessed by the Rating Scale are provided in Appendix B.

The Rating Scale is used to provide a picture of four general areas of each residential facility:

1. The overall site
2. Various aspects of the physical environment
3. The residents
4. The staff

Rate each feature of the facility or program according to the instructions.

Please fill in the information below

Date_____

Name of facility_____

Type of facility (e.g., nursing home, domiciliary, residential care facility, or senior citizens apartments) _____

How long has this facility been in operation? _____

Sponsoring agency or name of corporation _____

Your name _____

Section I: Ratings of the Overall Site
(Check the appropriate box)

1. As a *neighborhood* for living, how does the area around this site look?

   ☐ (3) Very pleasant and attractive

   ☐ (2) Mildly pleasant and attractive

   ☐ (1) Ordinary, perhaps even slightly unattractive

   1 ☐ (0) Unattractive, slum-like

2. How attractive are the site *grounds?*

   ☐ (3) Very attractive   Landscaping or very attractive natural growth; well maintained; no litter or weeds, clean paths, neatly trimmed

   ☐ (2) Somewhat attractive   Show signs of care and frequent maintenance

   ☐ (1) Ordinary   Ordinary looking or somewhat attractive but poorly maintained; little landscaping, some weeds or litter

   2 ☐ (0) Unattractive   No grounds, sidewalks only; show little or no maintenance

3. How attractive are the site *buildings?*

   ☐ (3) Very attractive   Unique and attractive design, excellent maintenance

   ☐ (2) Somewhat attractive   May show some deterioration on close inspection, or design is adequate but not unusually attractive

   ☐ (1) Ordinary   Buildings are somewhat attractive but poorly maintained, or are not notable in either design or maintenance

   3 ☐ (0) Unattractive   Buildings are deteriorated or unattractive

Section II: Ratings of
Environmental Characteristics

Part I: Ratings of Four Major Living Areas

    a. Lounge, commons room, living room

    b. Dining room

    c. Residents' bedrooms (or individual apartments)

    d. Hallways

Directions: Rate each of these four areas and enter your rating (0, 1, 2, 3) in the appropriate space.

   1. *Noise Level*

(3) Very quiet	Noticeable absence of sounds, even when area is being used by many residents
(2) Quiet	Some sounds present, but reading would be easy
(1) Somewhat noisy	Many sounds present or occasional loud interruptions
(0) Very noisy	Sounds are loud and distracting (e.g., sustained noise from buzzers, cleaning equipment, etc.)

_____Lounge   _____Dining room   _____Bedrooms   _____Hallways

    4   5   6   7

  2. *Odors*

(3) Fresh	Living spaces have pleasantly fresh odor
(2) No odors	Nothing noticeable about the air, "normal"
(1) Slightly objectionable	Air is slightly tainted in some way; stale, close, musty, medicinal
(0) Distinctly objectionable	Unpleasant odors are apparent

_____Lounge   _____Dining room   _____Bedrooms   _____Hallways

    8   9   10   11

3. *Level of Illumination*

    (3) Ample lighting   Brightly illuminated, but without glare; reading be easy in all areas of room

    (2) Good lighting   Lighting basically good, but may be low, uneven or glaring in some areas; reading easy in most areas of room

    (1) Barely adequate   Lighting is low, uneven, or glaring; reading is difficult in only certain areas of the room

    (0) Inadequate lighting   Illumination very low or very glaring in most areas of room; reading difficult

_____Lounge   _____Dining room   _____Bedrooms   _____Hallways
   12   13   14   15

4. *Cleanliness of Walls and Floors (or Rugs)*

    (3) Very clean   Both walls and floors are kept very clean, spotless; floors are polished

    (2) Clean   Both walls and floors are cleaned regularly; some dust in corners, fingerprints on walls

    (1) Somewhat dirty   Either walls or floors need cleaning; considerable dust, fingerprints or stains

    (0) Very dirty   Both walls and floors need a major cleaning; surfaces stained, scuff marks, surfaces dirty to the touch

42 _____Lounge   _____Dining room   _____Bedrooms   _____Hallways
      16   17   18   19

5. *Condition of Walls and Floors (or Rugs)*

    (3) Like new   Both walls and floors are new looking; appear recently installed or painted

    (2) Good condition   Good condition; either walls or floors show wear on close examination

    (1) Fair condition   Walls or floors show wear, but only in heavily used areas

    (0) Poor condition   Walls or floors show evident wear; worn spots, cracks, peeling, faded

_____Lounge   _____Dining room   _____Bedrooms   _____Hallways
   20   21   22   23

6. *Condition of Furniture*

    (3) Excellent condition   Like new; well kept, spotless, highly polished or without stains

    (2) Good condition   Not new, but in good condition; slightly worn, small scratches, dusty, a few stains, some dirt in creases

    (1) Fair condition   Older, but still structurally sound and kept moderately clean

    (0) Deteriorated   Old and in poor repair; some tears, stains, dirt or dust; may be structurally unsound or dangerous

_____Lounge   _____Dining room   _____Bedroom

   24   25   26

7. *Window Areas*

    (3) Many windows   Living space has large window areas that give an open feeling

    (2) Adequate windows   Windows are sufficient to allow good light; there is no closed-in feeling

    (1) Few windows   Room tends to be dark, even on sunny days; there is a feeling of being closed in

    (0) No windows   There are no windows, or the windows are not functional

_____Lounge   _____Dining room   _____Bedrooms

   27   28   29

8. *View From Windows—Interest*

    (3) Very interesting   View overlooks very interesting and continuous activities (e.g., children playing)

    (2) Interesting   View overlooks some activities that draw mild attention (e.g., pedestrians or cars passing)

    (1) Lacks interest   View is fairly dull or only rarely captures interest

    (0) No interest   Basically nothing happening; looking outside is boring

_____Lounge   _____Dining room   _____Bedrooms

   27   28   29   30

**Part II: Ratings of Residents'
Bedrooms or Apartments**
(Check the appropriate box)

9. *Variation in Design of
   Residents' Rooms (Apts.)*

   ☐ (3) Distinct variation   As if effort was made to vary style and
                                       decor from room to room

   ☐ (2) Moderate variation   Rooms (apartments) are distinct, but
                                       there is a general decor throughout

   ☐ (1) Nearly identical   Some variation in size, shape, or
                                       furniture arrangement; variation is not
                                       noticeable unless looked for

33 ☐ (0) Identical   No variation except for decorational
                                       detail such as paint or rug color

10. *Personalization of
    Residents' Rooms (Apts.)*

    ☐ (3) Much personalization   Most of the furnishings and objects in
                                        the room belong to the individual;
                                        time and energy have been spent in
                                        personalizing the rooms

    ☐ (2) Some personalization   Residents have added personal objects
                                        such as rugs, pictures, chairs, favorite
                                        objects

    ☐ (1) Little personalization   Some family pictures or personal
                                        articles, but room does not seem to
                                        "belong" to an individual

34 ☐ (0) No personalization
        is evident

Part III: Rating the Facility as a Whole
(Check the appropriate box)

11. *Distinctiveness of All Living Spaces*

☐ (3) Much distinctiveness   A concerted effort has been made to vary the decor from room to room

☐ (2) Moderate distinctiveness   Furnishings vary from room to room, but the overall room design is the same; wall texture and floor coverings show little variation

☐ (1) Some distinctiveness   Very little variation, even in furnishings; somewhat institutional, but some areas are distinct such as the lounge or lobby (e.g., floor coverings vary, pictures, or signs)

35   ☐ (0) little distinctiveness   Institutional appearance; most areas are quite similar, as in a hospital (without furniture, all rooms look about the same)

12. *Overall Pleasantness of the Facility*

☐ (3) Quite pleasant   "I would feel good about placing a person in this housing."

☐ (2) Pleasant   "I would not feel badly about placing a person in this housing if they were in some way limited to this choice (finances, closeness to friends, etc.)."

☐ (1) Somewhat unpleasant   "I would feel uneasy about placing a person here."

36   ☐ (0) Distinctly unpleasant   "I would not place a person here."

13. *Overall Attractiveness of the Facility*

☐ (3) Highly appealing — Attractive enough to be desirable for one's own home

☐ (2) Appealing — Overall effect is favorable; fairly comfortable, although there may be some drawbacks (old furnishings, inconvenient)

☐ (1) Neutral — Neither positive nor negative features especially stand out; ordinary

37 ☐ (0) Unattractive — Physical plant is unattractive or unappealing; it may be cold or somewhat sterile; arouses negative feelings

Section III: Ratings of Residents
(Check the appropriate box)

(Rate only those residents in the general living areas)

1. *Personal Grooming*

   ☐ (3) Very well-groomed — Appear well washed, hair looks combed, men are clean shaven

   ☐ (2) Fairly well-groomed — Neither distinctly clean nor dirty, appearance presentable

   ☐ (1) Not well-groomed — Hair looks uncombed or men unshaven, but appearance still satisfactory

   38 ☐ (0) Ungroomed or unclean — Hair, nails, beard, and so on look unattended and uncared for; unpleasant odors may be apparent

2. *Condition of Clothing*

   ☐ (3) Very neat and clean — Freshly laundered and pressed, in very good condition

   ☐ (2) Moderately neat and clean — Reasonably clean, although some clothes may be somewhat worn or wrinkled or both

   ☐ (1) Somewhat worn or soiled — May look somewhat worn or soiled, but appearance is still generally satisfactory

   39 ☐ (0) Generally worn or soiled — Generally soiled or wrinkled; disheveled appearance

3. *Interaction of Residents*

   ☐ (3) Considerable interaction — Majority of the residents seen are interacting; few isolates observed

   ☐ (2) Moderate interaction — About half of the residents seen are interacting or in close proximity to others

   ☐ (1) Some interaction — Some residents seen interacting in pairs or in small groups, but many are alone

   40 ☐ (0) Very little interaction — Most residents seen either walking or sitting alone or in bed

4. *Brief Verbal Exchanges* (greetings and pleasantries)

☐ (3) Many instances   Residents generally greet each other or exchange a few words when they meet or sit next to each other

☐ (2) Several instances   Residents sometimes greet each other and sometimes do not

☐ (1) Few instances   Some residents greet each other, but most seem to be withdrawn and isolated

41   ☐ (0) Very few instances   Residents generally seem withdrawn and unaware of one another

5. *General Amount of Activity*

☐ (3) Very high   Most residents seem busy or active most of the time (e.g., visiting, reading, playing cards)

☐ (2) High   Activity level seems high, but some residents are inactive

☐ (1) Moderate   Some residents seem moderately busy, but many are rather inactive

42   ☐ (0) Low   Few residents seem at all active

Section IV: Ratings of Staff

1. *Quality of Interaction*

☐ (3) Personal interaction   Staff interact with residents in a warm, personal manner

☐ (2) Warm professional interaction   Much of the staff's contact occurs as a part of their duties, but contact is personalized and informal

☐ (1) Formal professional interaction   Most contact is formal and relates mainly to duties

43   ☐ (0) Stern professional interaction   Contact is formal or abrupt; some condescension may be evident

2. *Physical Contact With Residents*

    ☐ (3) Considerable physical contact   Extended or intimate contact between residents and staff observed (e.g., prolonged resting of arm on shoulder)

    ☐ (2) Moderate physical contact   staff seen assisting residents walking or holding resident's hand or arm during conversation

    ☐ (1) Some physical contact   Resident may take a staff person's arm for assistance but little other physical contact observed

    ☐ (0) Little physical contact   Little or no physical contact observed

3. *Organization*

44   ☐ (3) Very well organized   Facility is very well organized; staff members perform duties efficiently; residents' needs are met promptly

    ☐ (2) Fairly well organized   Facility generally well organized, but some confusion or inefficiency evident in procedures or handling of residents' needs

    ☐ (1) Somewhat disorganized   Facility somewhat disorganized; residents' basic needs met, but residents may experience long delays; some tasks may remain undone

45   ☐ (0) Very disorganized   Facility appears quite disorganized and confusing; residents' basic needs may be poorly met

4. *Availability of Staff to Residents*

    ☐ (3) Nearly constant availability   Resident have almost constant access to staff; a staff member usually visible from the doorway of each room

    ☐ (2) Periodic availability   Residents usually have access to staff; staff members around much of the time; systematic checks of residents

    ☐ (1) Some availability   Staff members are around some of the time; usually residents must seek staff out

46   ☐ (0) Almost no availability   Residents must seek staff out and may have difficulty locating a staff member when the need arises

5. *Staff Conflict*

     ☐ (3) No conflict   Detected no evidence of conflict among staff members; staff members show signs of friendliness toward one another

     ☐ (2) Mild conflict   Mild uneasiness or tension observed in some staff interactions

     ☐ (1) Moderate conflict   Some problems observed in staff interaction (e.g., conflict some critical or disparaging comments may occur)

47   ☐ (0) Considerable conflict   Staff observed complaining to or about one another; some harshness, anger, or bad temper observed

BACKGROUND INFORMATION
FORM (BIF)

Name (optional)_____Today's date_____ 1-2

Sex   1 ☐ Male   2 ☐ Female   3

We would like you to answer a few questions about your background.

1. In what year were you born?_____   3

2. Were you born in the United States? .... 1 ☐ Yes   2 ☐ No   6

3. Are you fluent in a language other than English? .... 1 ☐ Yes   2 ☐ No   7

   If so, what language?_____   8

4. What is your ethnic background? (Check one)

   1 ☐ Asian or Asian American   4 ☐ White

   2 ☐ Black or African American   5 ☐ Other

   3 ☐ Latino or Hispanic   9

5. What is your religious preference?_____   10

6. What is your marital status? (Check one)

   1 ☐ Married   3 ☐ Separated or divorced

   2 ☐ Widowed   4 ☐ Single

7. How much schooling did you complete?_____   11

8. What was your major occupation?_____   14-16

9. Do you presently receive Medicaid (*not* Medicare)   1   2   17
   or supplemental Security Income (SSI)? .... ☐ Yes   ☐ No

10. How long have you lived at your present address?_____   18

11. How much help do you need with the following activities?
    (Check the box that indicates how much help you need.)

	No help needed	*Some help needed*	*Cannot do at all*
	1	2	3
a. Taking care of my appearance (e.g., combing my hair or shaving)	☐	☐	☐ 20
b. Eating meals	☐	☐	☐
c. Dressing and undressing	☐	☐	☐
d. Walking	☐	☐	☐
e. Getting in and out of bed	☐	☐	☐
f. Bathing or showering	☐	☐	☐ 25
g. Handling my money (paying bills)	☐	☐	☐
h. Using the telephone	☐	☐	☐
i. Going shopping	☐	☐	☐

                                                            1   2

12. Do you presently use a prescribed medication? ☐ Yes ☐ No

13. Do you have trouble seeing to read (even with glasses)? ☐ Yes ☐ No

14. Do you (or should you) use a hearing aid? ☐ Yes ☐ No

15. Put a check next to all of the activities you have done during the past week.

_____Watched TV

_____Listened to music

_____Read a newspaper or book

_____Wrote (letters, poems, etc.)

_____Sewed or knitted

_____Played cards, checkers, chess, or a similar game

_____Played pool, bingo, or dominoes

_____Drew or painted

_____Engaged in photography, woodworking, ceramics, or another hobby

_____Took care of plants or gardened

_____Visited with other residents

_____Went outside

_____Went for a walk   32-49

16. On the average, how often do you get out for the following activities? For each activity, put a check in the box that best describes how often you go out to participate in that activity.

	Rarely or never	A few times a year	Once or twice a month	Once a week or more
	1	2	3	4
Visit friends or relatives	☐	☐	☐	☐ 45
Go on a ride or tour	☐	☐	☐	☐
Go to a sports event	☐	☐	☐	☐
Go on a picnic	☐	☐	☐	☐
Attend religious services	☐	☐	☐	☐
Attend a funeral or memorial service	☐	☐	☐	☐ 50
Go shopping	☐	☐	☐	☐
Eat in a restaurant	☐	☐	☐	☐
Attend a concert or play	☐	☐	☐	☐
Attend a movie	☐	☐	☐	☐
Go to a party	☐	☐	☐	☐ 55
Engage in volunteer or paid work	☐	☐	☐	☐
Go on an overnight trip	☐	☐	☐	☐
Go to a senior citizens center	☐	☐	☐	☐ 58

17. On the average, how often do you participate in the following activities offered here?

	Rarely or never	A few times a year	Once or twice a month	Once a week or more
	1	2	3	4
Exercise or fitness activity	☐	☐	☐	☐59
Outside entertainment (e.g., pianist or singer)	☐	☐	☐	☐
Discussion group	☐	☐	☐	☐
Reality orientation group	☐	☐	☐	☐
Self-help or mutual support group	☐	☐	☐	☐
Film or movie	☐	☐	☐	☐
Club, social group, drama, or singing group	☐	☐	☐	☐65
Class or lecture	☐	☐	☐	☐
Bingo, cards, or other game	☐	☐	☐	☐
Party	☐	☐	☐	☐
Religious service	☐	☐	☐	☐
Social hour (e.g., coffee or cocktail hour)	☐	☐	☐	☐
Arts and crafts	☐	☐	☐	☐71

Appendix B:
Hand-Scoring Worksheets

RESIDENT AND STAFF
INFORMATION FORM (RESIF)

Before scoring the RESIF, be sure that all relevant information has been converted to percentage of total residents or staff. Transfer the information from the RESIF as indicated and perform necessary computations. (Section and item number are indicated for each question.) Circle "M" if information is missing.

1. Resident Social Resources

NOTE: Do not score this dimension if any item is missing.

Section I   Percentage

  6. What percentage of the residents are married? .... M _____

  7. What percentage have more than an eighth-grade
     education? .... M _____

  8. What percentage of the residents are semiprofessional,
     managerial, professional or executives? .... M _____

 12. What percentage of the residents do not receive
     Medicaid or SSI (whichever is applicable)? .... M _____

SCORING: Add the numbers in the percentage column and enter the sum as the total score. To compute the percentage score, divide the total score by 4.

$$\underline{\hspace{2cm}} \div 4 = \underline{\hspace{3cm}}$$
   (total score)   (percentage score)

236

2. *Resident Heterogeneity*

Section I   Score

2. Are between 30% and 70% of the residents male?........ M Yes No _____

3. Do at least four of the five age categories have 5%
   or more of the residents?... M Yes No _____

4. What percentage of the residents are

   _____% Asian American   _____% White

   _____% Black   _____% Other

   _____% Hispanic

   Put a check next to each category that contains
   1% or more of the residents. Put a circle around
   each category that contains 5% or more of the
   residents. Are at least three categories checked
   and at least two categories circled? .... M Yes No _____

5. Do at least three of the five religious background
   categories have 5% or more of the residents? .... M Yes No _____

6. Do at least three of the four marital status
   categories have 10% or more of the residents? .... M Yes No _____

7. Do at least four of the six educational categories
   have 5% or more of the residents? .... M Yes No _____

8. Do at least five of the seven occupational
   categories have 5% or more of the residents? .... M Yes No _____

9. Were 10% or more of the residents born outside
   the United States? .... M Yes No _____

11. Do residents speak at least two languages other
    than English? .... M Yes No _____

    Do 10% or more of the residents speak a language
    other than English? .... M Yes No _____

SCORING: For each "yes" that has been circled, put a "1" in the score column. For each M that has been circled, put an M in the score column. Otherwise, put a "0" in the score column. Add the numbers in the score column and enter the sum as the total score. To obtain the total points possible, subtract the total number of Ms from 10. To compute the percentage score, divide the total score by the total points possible and multiply by 100.

_____ ÷ _____ × 100 = _____

(total score)   (total points possible)   (percentage score)

3. Resident Functional Abilities

Section II, Part I   Percentage

What percentage of the residents

   1. can take care of their own appearance ....M _____

   2. can eat their meals without any help ....M _____

   3. can dress and undress themselves ....M _____

   4. can walk without any help...M _____

   5. can get in and out of bed without any help ....M _____

   6. can take a bath or shower without any help...........................M _____

   7. can get to the bathroom on time ....M _____

   8. can make their needs or wishes clearly understood................M _____

   9. can handle their own money ....M _____

  10. can use the telephone without any help ....M _____

  11. can go shopping for groceries and clothes
      without any help ....M _____

Section II, Part II

   1. are *not* on a prescribed medication?.......................................M _____

   2. can *see* well enough to read? ....M _____

   3. do *not* need a hearing aid? ....M _____

   4. know what day and year it is? ....M _____

SCORING: Add the numbers in the percentage column and enter the sum as the total score. To obtain the total points possible, subtract the total number of Ms from 15. To compute the percentage score, divide the total score by the total points possible.

        _____ ÷ _____ = _____

       (total score) (total points possible)   (percentage score)

4. Resident Activity Level

Section II, Part III   Percentage

During the past week, how many residents
have taken part in these activities?

1. Watched TV ....M _____

2. Listened to music...M _____

3. Read a newspaper or book ....M _____

4. Wrote ....M _____

5. Sewed or knitted...M _____

6. Played cards, checkers, chess, or a similar game.....................M _____

7. Played pool, bingo, or dominoes...M _____

8. Drew or painted ....M _____

9. Engaged in photography, woodworking,
   ceramics, or hobby ....M _____

10. Took care of plants or gardened ....M _____

11. Visited with other residents...M _____

12. Went outside on a nice day ....M _____

13. Took a walk...M _____

SCORING: Add the numbers in the percentage column and enter the sum as the total score. To obtain the total points possible, subtract the total number of Ms from 13. To compute the percentage score, divide the total score by the total points possible.

_____ ÷ _____ = _____

(total score)   (total points possible)   (percentage score)

5. Resident Activities in the Community

Section III   Percentage

How many residents leave the facility for these
activities *at least a few times a year?*

1. To visit friends or relatives .... M _____
2. To go on a ride or tour .... M _____
3. To go to a ball game or other sports event .... M _____
4. To go on a picnic .... M _____
5. To attend religious services .... M _____
6. To attend a funeral or memorial service .... M _____
7. To go shopping .... M _____
8. To eat in a restaurant .... M _____
9. To attend a concert or play .... M _____
10. To attend the movies .... M _____
11. To go to parties .... M _____
12. To engage in volunteer or paid work .... M _____
13. To go on an overnight trip .... M _____
14. To go to a senior citizens center .... M _____

**SCORING: Add the numbers in the percentage column and enter the sum as the
total score. To obtain the total points possible, subtract the total number of Ms
from 14. To compute the percentage score, divide the total score by the total
points possible.**

$$\underline{\hspace{2cm}} \div \underline{\hspace{3cm}} = \underline{\hspace{3cm}}$$

(total score)   (total points possible)   (percentage score)

6. *Staff Resources*

Section IV, Part I   Score

1. Are there some hours for *both* physicians
   and occupational/physical therapists?........................... M Yes No _____

1. Are there some hours for psychologists, psychiatrists,
   social workers, clergymen, or religious counselors? ...... M Yes No _____

1. Are there some hours for *both* activity directors/
   recreational therapists *and* nutritionists/dietitians? .... M Yes No _____

3. Have 50% or more of the staff worked in the
   facility more than 12 months?.................................... M Yes No _____

4. What percentage of the present staff members are

   _____% male 18-30   _____% female 18-30

   _____% male 31-40   _____% female 31-40

   _____% male 41-50   _____% female 41-50

   _____% male 51 and over   _____% female 51 and over

   Do six of these eight categories have at least
   some staff in them? .... M Yes No _____

   Are 1% or more of the staff members
   "male 51 and over?"....................................... M Yes No _____

   Are 10% or more of the staff members
   "female 51 and over?".................................... M Yes No _____

   5a. Do staff members who give direct services speak
       at least two languages other than English?............ M Yes No _____

       Do 10% or more of the staff fluently speak a
       language other than English? .... M Yes No _____

6. Is there an in-service training program? .... M Yes No _____

   6a. Is the in-service training program "at regular staff
       meetings on a continuing basis" or "at regularly
       scheduled meetings with special programs?" .... M Yes No _____

Section IV, Part II

  2. Is the number of "volunteer hours/month/resident"
      greater than or equal to 1? .... M Yes No _____

4 × _____ ÷ _____ = _____

     (volunteer hr/week)   (No. of residents)   (volunteer hr/mo/resident)

    3a. Is the volunteer training program "ongoing,
        regular meetings" or "regularly scheduled
        meetings with special programs"? .... M Yes No _____

**SCORING: For each yes that has been circled, put a 1 in the score column. For
each M that has been circled, put an M in the score column. Otherwise, put a 0
in the score column. Add the numbers in the score column and enter the sum as
the total score. To obtain the total points possible, subtract the total number of
Ms from 13. To compute the percentage score, divide the total score by the total
points possible and multiply by 100.**

_____ ÷ _____ × 100 = _____

    (total score) (total points possible)   (percentage score)

PHYSICAL AND ARCHITECTURAL
FEATURES CHECKLIST (PAF)

Transfer the information from the PAF by circling the answer. (Section and item number are indicated for each question.)

1. *Community Accessibility*

Section I   Score

5. Are the following community resources located
   within easy walking distance of the facility (1/4 mile)?

   5a. Grocery store..Yes No _____

   5b. Drugstore ....Yes No _____

   5c. Senior citizens center...Yes No _____

   5d. Movie theater ....Yes No _____

   5e. Church or synagogue..Yes No _____

   5f. Public library ....Yes No _____

   5g. Bank ....Yes No _____

   5h. Hospital...Yes No _____

   5i. Doctor's office...Yes No _____

   5j. Dentist's office..Yes No _____

   5k. Post office...Yes No _____

   5l. Park ....Yes No _____

6. Does the city or town within which this facility
   is located have a public transportation system?.................Yes No _____

7. Is there a public transportation stop within easy
   walking distance (1/4 mile)? ....Yes No _____

   7a. If so, does it have benches? ....Yes No _____

8. Are there lights in the surrounding streets? ....Yes No _____

SCORING: For each yes that has been circled, put a 1 in the score column. Otherwise, put a 0 in the score column. Add the numbers in the score column and enter the sum as the total score. To compute the percentage score, divide the total score by 16 and multiply by 100.

_____ ÷ 16 × 100 = _____

(total score)   (percentage score)

2. *Physical Amenities*

Section II   Score

   1. Is the main entrance sheltered from sun and rain? .... Yes No _____

   4c. Is the seating in front of the building
       protected from weather? .... Yes No _____

   6b. Are umbrella tables available? .... Yes No _____

   6c. Is the outdoor furniture in good condition? .... Yes No _____

   6d. Is there a covered area (rainproof)? .... Yes No_____

   6e. Is there an area with a sunscreen or
       protection from the sun? .... Yes No _____

   8. Is there a lawn? .... Yes No _____

Section III, Part II

   4. Are the halls decorated? .... Yes No _____

   5. Are there drinking fountains? .... Yes No _____

   5a. Is there at least one drinking fountain on each floor? .. Yes No _____

   6. Are there public telephones? .... Yes No _____

   6a. Is there at least one public telephone on each floor? .... Yes No _____

   6b. Is there a writing surface by the telephone? .... Yes No _____

Section III, Part III

   6. Are there any table lamps? .... Yes No _____

Section III, Part VII

   6. Is there an air-conditioning system? .... Yes No _____

   7. Is there a chapel or meditation room? .... Yes No _____

   8. Is there a gift shop, commissary, or store? .... Yes No _____

   11a. Are the vending machines used by residents? .... Yes No _____

   12. Is there a laundry area for residents' use? .... Yes No _____

Section III, Part VIII

   6. Are there mirrors in the bathrooms? .... All Some None _____

   13. Does each resident have access to both a
       bathtub and shower? .... Yes No ____

Section III, Part IX

    4. Is there wall space on which residents can
       hang pictures? ....All Some None ____

    5. Is there adequate light for reading? ....All Some None ____

    6. Is there a mirror? ....All Some None ____

    7. Is there a window sill that is wide enough
       for flowers? ....All Some None ____

    8. Are the floors a light color? ....All Some None ____

    9. Are the walls a light color? ....All Some None ____

  10. Are there individual heating controls? ....All Some None ____

  11. Are there individual air-conditioning controls? ....All Some None ____

  17. Do all the apartments have their own kitchen or kitchenette?
      OR

Section III, Part VII

    9. Is there a kitchen area in which a resident or
       visitor can make a cup of coffee, heat some soup,
       or the like? ....Yes No ____

SCORING: For each yes or all that has been circled, put a 1 in the score column. Otherwise, put a 0 in the score column. Add the numbers in the score column and enter the sum as the total score. To compute the percentage score, divide the total score by 30 and multiply by 100.

$$\underline{\hspace{3cm}} \div 30 \times 100 = \underline{\hspace{4cm}}$$

    (total score)   (percentage score)

3. Social-Recreational Aids

Section II   Score

    4. Is there outside seating in the front of the building? .... Yes No _____

    4d. Does it provide a view of pedestrians and
         other activity? .... Yes No _____

    5. Is there a patio or open courtyard? .... Yes No _____

    6a. Are tables available? .... Yes No _____

    6f. Is there a barbecue? .... Yes No _____

    6g. Is there a shuffleboard game area? .... Yes No _____

    7. Is there a garden area for resident use? .... Yes No _____

    11. Is there parking for visitors? .... Yes No _____

Section III, Part I

    12. Is there seating in the lobby? .... Yes No _____

    13a. Is the entrance lounge furnished for resting
        or conversation? .... Yes No _____

Section III, Part III

    2. Are any lounges near an entrance or traveled hallway? ...... Yes No _____

    3. Are there writing desks or tables? .... Yes No _____

    4. Are there small tables for socializing or playing games? ..... Yes No _____

    5. Is reading material available on tables or shelves? .... Yes No _____

    8. Is there a quiet lounge with no television? .... Yes No _____

Section III, Part III and Section III, Part IV

    1a. How many lounges are there? _____

    1a. How many special activity areas are there? _____

    All together is there more than one lounges and
    special activity areas? .... Yes No _____

Section III, Part IV

   2. Is there a library from which books can be borrowed? ...... Yes No _____

   3. Is there a music or listening room? .... Yes No _____

   4. Pool or billiard table? .... Yes No _____

   5. Ping-pong table? .... Yes No _____

   6. Piano or organ? .... Yes No _____

   7. One or more television sets? .... Yes No _____

   8. One or more phonographs? .... Yes No _____

   9. One or more radios? .... Yes No _____

  10. One or more sewing machines? .... Yes No _____

Section III, Part V

   2. Are there small tables which seat fewer than six? *AND*

   3. Are there large tables which seat more than six? .... Yes No _____

Section III, Part VII

  10. Is there a snack bar? .... Yes No _____

Section III, Part IX

  12. Is there a telephone or a telephone
      connection? .... All Some None _____

SCORING: For each yes or all that has been circled, put a 1 in the score column. Otherwise, put a 0 in the score column. Add the numbers in the score column and enter the sum as the total score. To compute the percentage score, divide the total score by 28 and multiply by 100.

      _____ ÷ 28 × 100 = _____

      (total score)   (percentage score)

4. *Prosthetic Aids*

Section II   Score

  9. Is there parking reserved for handicapped? .... Yes No _____

Section III, Part I

  1. Can one enter the building without having to
     use any stairs? .... Yes No _____

  5. Does the front door open automatically? .... Yes No _____

  6. Does the front door swing closed by itself? .... Yes No _____

  7. Is the front door wide enough for a wheelchair? .... Yes No _____

Section III, Part II

  1. Are the hallways 8 feet wide or wider? .... Yes No _____

  3. Are there handrails in the halls? .... Yes No _____

    5b. Are the drinking fountains accessible to
       wheelchair residents? .... Yes No _____

    6c. Are public telephones accessible to wheelchair
       residents? .... Yes No _____

    6d. Does at least one telephone have a loudness control
       in the receiver for people who are hard of hearing? .. Yes No _____

Section III, Part III

  7. Is the furniture spaced wide enough for wheelchairs? .... Yes No _____

Section III, Part V

  4. Is aisle space between tables at least 60 inches? .... Yes No _____

Section III, Part VIII

  2. Do the bathroom doors open out? .... All Some None _____

  3. Are there handrails or safety bars? .... All Some None _____

  4. Are there lift bars next to the toilet? .... All Some None _____

  9. Is there turning radius for a wheelchair
     (5 feet × 5 feet)? .... All Some None _____

    13c. Is there a flexible shower? .... Yes No _____

    13d. Is there a seat included in the shower? .... Yes No _____

    13e. Is a wheelchair-entered shower available? .... Yes No _____

Section III, Part IX

13. Is there room for wheelchair use? ....All Some None _____

14. Are there handrails?...All Some None _____

STEP 1: For each yes or "all" that has been circled, put a 1 in the score column. Otherwise, put a 0 in the score column.

Section III, Part II

8. Does a resident have to climb any steps to have access
   to all areas of the building intended for resident use? ....Yes No _____

Section III, Part VIII

1. Are there raised thresholds at the entrances? ....All Some None _____

5. Are the towel racks and dispensers higher than
   40 inches from the floor? ....All Some None _____

STEP 2: For each no or "none" that has been circled, put a 1 in the score column. Otherwise, put a 0 in the score column.

SCORING: Add the numbers in the score column and enter the sum as the total score. To compute the percentage score, divide the total score by 24 and multiply by 100.

_____ ÷ 24 × 100 = _____

   (total score)   (percentage score)

5. Orientational Aids

Section III, Part I   Score

  4. Are written instructions posted outside that explain
     how to get in if the front door is locked? .... Yes No _____

  9. Is there a reception area or reception desk? .... Yes No _____

 15. Is there a large face clock in the lobby/entrance area? .... Yes No _____

Section III, Part II

 11. Is each floor or corridor color coded or numbered? .... Yes No _____

 12. Are the residents' names on or next to their doors? .... Yes No _____

 13. Is it easy for new residents to find their way around? .... Yes No _____

Section III, Part VII

  1. Is there a map of community resources in
     a public location? .... Yes No _____

  2. Is there a bulletin board in a public location? .... Yes No _____

  3. Is there a posted list of the staff? .... Yes No _____

    3a. If so, does it include pictures? .... Yes No _____

  4. Is there a posted list of residents? .... Yes No _____

    4a. If so, does it include pictures? .... Yes No _____

  5. Is there a sound system or public address system? .... Yes No _____

SCORING: For each yes that has been circled, put a 1 in the score column. Otherwise, put a 0 in the score column. Add the numbers in the score column and enter the sum as the total score. To compute the percentage score, divide the total score by 13 and multiply by 100.

       _____ ÷ 13 × 100 = _____

        (total score)   (percentage score)

6. Safety Features

Section II   Score

2. Is the outside building area well lighted?.............................Yes No _____

3a. Are the outside walk and entrance visible from the
lobby or ground floor social space? ....Yes No _____

3b. Are the outside walk and entrance visible from
the office or station of an employee?...........................Yes No _____

4a. Is the outside seating in front of the building visible
from the lobby or ground floor social space?
(n.a. if there is no outside seating in front.)............n.a. Yes No _____

4b. Is the outside seating in front of the building
visible from the office or station of an employee?
(n.a. if there is no outside seating in front.)............n.a. Yes No _____

Section III, Part I

2. Is the entry from outside limited to one unlocked door? ...Yes No _____

3. Is there a bell or call system outside?..................................Yes No _____

8. Is there someone who usually monitors access
to the building? ....Yes No _____

10. Is there a place for visitors to sign in? ....Yes No _____

14. Can one see into the lobby or entrance area from
a lounge or other ground floor social space?.....................Yes No _____

Section III, Part II

7. Are there smoke detection devices in the halls?..................Yes No _____

9. Are the stairs well lighted?
(n.a. if there are no stairs.) ....n.a. Yes No _____

10. Are there nonskid surfaces on stairs and ramps?
(n.a. if there are no stairs or ramps.) ....n.a. Yes No _____

Section III, Part VIII

7. Are there nonslip surfaces in areas subject
to wetness? ....All Some None _____

8. Are there call buttons in the bathrooms?..............All Some None _____

Section III, Part IX

   15. Are there smoke detection devices?.......................All Some None _____

   16. Is there a call button or telephone connection
       in every room? ....All Some None _____

STEP 1: For each yes or "all" that has been circled, put a 1 in the score column. For each n.a. that has been circled, write n.a. in the score column. Otherwise, put a 0 in the score column.

Section III, Part II

   2. Are the hallways crowded or are there obstructions?.........Yes No _____

STEP 2: If no has been circled, put a 1 in the score column. Otherwise, put a 0 in the score column.

SCORING: Add the numbers in the score column and enter the sum as the total score. Count the number of n.a.s in the score column. To obtain the total points possible, subtract the total number of n.a.s from 18. To compute the percentage score, divide the total score by the total points possible and multiply by 100.

     _____ ÷ _____ × 100 = _____

     (total score)   (total points possible)   (percentage score)

7. *Staff Facilities*

Section II   Score

  10. Is there parking for staff? .... Yes No _____

Section III, Part VI

  2. Is there office space for the secretarial and clerical staff?... Yes No _____

  3. Are there offices for social service and counseling staff?.... Yes No _____

  4. Is there additional office space available for other staff?.... Yes No _____

  5. Are the offices free of distractions from
     adjacent activities?... Yes No _____

  6. Is there a separate room for handling mail,
     copying, or printing?... Yes No _____

  7. Is there a conference room? .... Yes No _____

  8. Is there a staff lounge?.. Yes No _____

    8a. If so, does it have tables? .... Yes No _____

    8b. Does it have comfortable chairs?................................. Yes No _____

    8c. Is the square feet per staff greater than
       or equal to 5? .... Yes No _____

_____ ÷ _____ = _____

(sq. ft. lounge)   (No. of staff FTEs)   (sq. ft. per staff)

SCORING: For each yes that has been circled, put a 1 in the score column. Otherwise, put a 0 in the score column. Add the numbers in the score column and enter the sum as the total score. To compute the percentage score, divide the total score by 11 and multiply by 100.

_____ ÷ 11 × 100 = _____

(total score)   (percentage score)

8. *Space Availability*

STEP 1: Perform the calculations as indicated. Compare the result with the cutoff point and circle the appropriate answer.

Section II   Score

12. Is the acreage per 100 residents
    greater than or equal to 4? .... Yes No _____

    _____ ÷ _____ × 100 = _____
    (acreage)   (No. residents)   (acres per 100 residents)

Section III, Part I

11a. Is the lobby's square footage per resident
     greater than or equal to 4? .... Yes No _____

     _____ ÷ _____ = _____
     (sq. ft.—lobby) (No. residents)   (sq. ft. per resident)

Section III, Part III

1a. Are the lounges per 40 residents greater
    than or equal to 1? .... Yes No _____

    _____ ÷ _____ × 40 = _____
    (No. lounges) (No. residents)   (lounges per 40 residents)

1d. Is the square footage per resident of the lounges
    greater than or equal to 10? .... Yes No _____

    _____ ÷ _____ = _____
    (total sq. ft.—lounges) (No. residents)   (sq. ft. per resident)

Section III, Part IV

1a. Are the special activity areas per 100 residents
    greater than or equal to 1? .... Yes No _____

    _____ ÷ _____ × 100 = _____
    (No. activity areas)   (No. residents)   (areas per 100 residents)

1d. Is the square footage per resident of special activity
    areas greater than or equal to 4? .... Yes No _____

    _____ ÷ _____ = _____
    (total sq. ft.—activity areas)   (No. residents)   (sq. ft. per resident)

Section III, Part V

1a. Are the dining rooms per 100 residents
greater than or equal to 1? ....Yes No _____

_____ ÷ _____ × 100 = _____
(No. dining rooms)   (No. residents)   (rooms per 100 residents)

1d. Is the square footage per resident of dining rooms
greater than or equal to 10? ....Yes No _____

_____ ÷ _____ = _____
(total sq. ft.—dining)   (No. residents)   (sq. ft. per resident)

Section III, Part VIII

10. Is the smallest bathroom 30 square feet or larger? ....Yes No _____

11. Is the largest bathroom square feet per resident greater
than or equal to 15? ....Yes No _____

_____ ÷ _____ = _____
(sq. ft.—largest bath)   (No. residents sharing)   (sq. ft. per resident)

Section III, Part IX

1. Is the average size per resident of rooms or apartments
greater than or equal to 150 square feet?..........................Yes No _____

_____ ÷ _____ = _____
(No. residents)   (No. rooms or apts.)   (average no. residents per room)

(_____ + _____) ÷ 2 = _____
(size smallest room)   (size largest room)   (average room size)

_____ ÷ _____ = _____
(average room size)   (average no.   (average size)
                        residents per room)   per resident

3. Is the square footage per resident for the largest room
or apartment greater than or equal to 100? ....Yes No _____

_____ ÷ _____ = _____
(size largest room)   (largest no. sharing)   (sq. ft. per resident)

20. Is the smallest per person closet area greater than or
    equal to 10 square feet? ....Yes No _____

**SCORING: For each yes that has been circled, put a 1 in the score column.
Otherwise, put a 0 in the score column. Add the numbers in the score column
and enter the sum as the total score. To compute the percentage score, divide the
total score by 13 and multiply by 100.**

_____ ÷ 13 × 100 = _____

   (total score)   (percentage score)

POLICY AND PROGRAM
INFORMATION FORM (POLIF)

Transfer the information from the POLIF by circling the answer or checking the correct box (section and item number are indicated for each question).

1. *Expectations for Functioning*

Section III, Part III

What is the policy with respect to the following behaviors and activities?

	Allowed/ Tolerated	Discouraged/ Intolerable	Score
1. Inability to make one's own bed	☐	☐	_____
2. Inability to clean one's own room	☐	☐	_____
3. Inability to feed oneself	☐	☐	_____
4. Inability to bathe or clean oneself	☐	☐	_____
5. Inability to dress oneself	☐	☐	_____
6. Incontinence	☐	☐	_____
7. Confusion or disorientation	☐	☐	_____
8. Depression	☐	☐	_____

STEP 1: For each "discouraged" or "intolerable" that has been checked, put a 1 in the score column. Otherwise, put a 0 in the score column.

Section I

4. Must a prospective resident be ambulatory? .... Yes No _____

STEP 2: If yes has been circled, put a 1 in the score column. Otherwise, put a 0 in the score column.

Section IV, Part II

   6. Does a staff member take attendance or count
      residents at mealtimes? .... Yes No _____

   11. Does the staff take a count or make a check each
       day to be sure that none of the residents are missing? .... Yes No _____

STEP 3: For each no that has been circled, put a 1 in the score column. Otherwise, put a 0 in the score column.

SCORING: Add the numbers in the score column and enter the sum as the total score. To compute the percentage score, divide the total score by 11 and multiply by 100.

$$\underline{\hspace{3cm}} \div 11 \times 100 = \underline{\hspace{3cm}}$$

   (total score)   (percentage score)

2. Acceptance of Problem Behavior

Section III, Part IV (p. 000)

What are the rules related to the following "problem" behaviors?

	Allowed/ Tolerated	Discouraged/ Intolerable	Score
1. Refusing to participate in programmed activities .... ☐	☐		_____
2. Refusing to take prescribed medicine .... ☐	☐		_____
3. Taking medicine other than that which is prescribed...................... ☐	☐		_____

STEP 1: For each "allowed" or "tolerated" that has been checked, put a 1 in the score column. Otherwise, put a 0 in the score column.

Section III, Part IV

What are the rules related to the following problem behaviors?

	Allowed Tolerated or Discouraged	*Intolerable*	*Score*
4. Taking too much medicine	☐	☐	_____
5. Being drunk	☐	☐	_____
6. Wandering around the building or grounds at night	☐	☐	_____
7. Leaving the building during the evening without letting anyone know	☐	☐	_____
8. Refusing to bathe or clean oneself regularly	☐	☐	_____
9. Creating a disturbance; being noisy or boisterous	☐	☐	_____
10. Pilfering or stealing others' belongings	☐	☐	_____
11. Damaging or destroying property	☐	☐	_____
12. Verbally threatening another resident	☐	☐	_____
13. Physically attacking another resident	☐	☐	_____
14. Physically attacking a staff member	☐	☐	_____
15. Attempting suicide	☐	☐	_____
16. Indecently exposing self	☐	☐	_____

STEP 2: For each allowed, tolerated, or discouraged that has been checked, put a 1 in the score column. Otherwise, put a 0 in the score column.

SCORING: Add the numbers in the score column and enter the sum as the total score. To compute the percentage score, divide the total score by 16 and multiply by 100.

$$\underline{\hspace{3cm}} \div 16 \times 100 = \underline{\hspace{4cm}}$$

     (total score)   (percentage score)

3. Policy Choice

(Mark n.a. if meal is not served.)
Section IV, Part II   Score

   1a. Is there at least an hour's range during which
      residents can choose to eat breakfast? ....n.a. Yes No _____

   2a. Is there at least an hour's range during
      which residents can choose to eat lunch? ....n.a. Yes No _____

   3a. Is there at least an hour's range during which
      residents can choose to eat dinner? ....n.a. Yes No _____

   5. Can residents choose to sit wherever
      they want at meals? ....n.a. Yes No _____

 13a. Do the rules allow for 11 hours or
      more of visiting per day? ....Yes No _____

STEP 1: For each yes that has been circled, put a 1 in the score column. For each n.a. that has been circled, write n.a. in the score column. Otherwise, put a 0 in the score column.

Section III, Part II

What is the policy with respect to the following personal possessions and behaviors?

	Allowed/ Tolerated	Discouraged/ Intolerable	Score
1. Drinking liquor in one's room............☐	☐	_____
2. Having one's own furniture in room...☐	☐	_____
3. Moving furniture around in room.......☐	☐	_____
4. Keeping a fish or bird in room ....☐	☐	_____
5. Keeping a hot plate or coffee maker in room....................................☐	☐	_____
6. Doing some laundry in the bathroom...☐	☐	_____
7. Drinking a glass of wine or beer at meals.......................................☐	☐	_____
8. Skipping breakfast to sleep late ....☐	☐	_____

STEP 2: For each encouraged or allowed that has been checked, put a 1 in the score column. Otherwise, put a 0 in the score column.

Section IV, Part II

    7. Is there a set time at which residents are awakened? .... Yes No ____

    8. Are there set times for baths or showers? .... Yes No ____

    9. Is there a set time for residents to go to bed at night? .... Yes No ____

  10. Is there a "curfew"? .... Yes No ____

  12. Are some building areas closed to residents at times? .... Yes No ____

  15. Is background music played in the building? .... Yes No ____

STEP 3: For each no that has been circled, put a 1 in the score column. Otherwise, put a 0 in the score column.

SCORING: Add the numbers in the score column and enter the sum as the total score. To obtain the number of points possible, subtract the total number of n.a.s from 19. To compute the percentage score, divide the total score by the total points possible and multiply by 100.

       _____ ÷ _____ × 100 = _____

      (total score)   (total points possible)   (percentage score)

4. *Resident Control*

Section III, Part V   Score

1. Are any of the residents paid for jobs
   within the facility?...Yes No _____

2. Do any of the residents have other types
   of chores or duties (unpaid) that they perform here?.........Yes No _____

   2a. Do 10% or more of the residents participate
   in chores or duties?...Yes No _____

3. Is there a residents' council?...Yes No _____

   3a. Are 4% or more of the residents on the
   residents' council?...Yes No _____

   3b. Does the residents' council meet twice a
   month or more?...Yes No _____

4. Are there regular "house meetings" for residents? ....Yes No _____

   4a. Do the house meetings occur once a month
   or more? ....Yes No _____

5. Are there resident committees? ....Yes No _____

   5a. Are 10% or more of the residents on committees? ......Yes No _____

   5a. Are there two or more committees that meet at
   least once a month? ....Yes No _____

   6b. Is there a newsletter that is primarily written
   by residents? ....Yes No _____

   7a. Is there a bulletin board being used by residents? ....Yes No _____

STEP 1: For each yes that has been circled, put a 1 in the score column. Otherwise, put a 0 in the score column.

Section III, Part VI

To what extent are residents involved in policymaking in the following areas?

1 = Staff/administrators basically decide by themselves

2 = Staff/administrators decide, but residents have input

3 = Residents decide, but staff has input

4 = Residents decide by themselves

	1 or 2	3 or 4	Score
1. Planning entertainment	☐	☐	_____
2. Planning educational activities.............	☐	☐	_____
3. Planning welcoming or orientation activities	☐	☐	_____
4. Deciding what kinds of new activities or programs will occur	☐	☐	_____
5. Making rules about attendance at activities	☐	☐	_____

STEP 2: For each "3" or "4" that has been checked, put a 1 in the score column. Otherwise, put a 0 in the score column.

To what extent are residents involved in policymaking in the following areas?

	1	2, 3, or 4	Score
6. Planning daily or weekly menus	☐	☐	_____
7. Setting mealtimes................................	☐	☐	_____
8. Setting visitors' hours	☐	☐	_____
9. Deciding on the decor of public areas...	☐	☐	_____
10. Dealing with safety hazards	☐	☐	_____
11. Dealing with residents' complaints......	☐	☐	_____
12. Making rules about the use of alcohol	☐	☐	_____

	1	2, 3, or 4	Score
13. Selecting new residents	☐	☐	____
14. Moving a resident from one bed or room to another	☐	☐	____
15. Deciding when a troublesome or sick resident will be asked to leave	☐	☐	____
16. Changes in staff	☐	☐	____

STEP 3: For each 2, 3, or 4 that has been checked, put a 1 in the score column. Otherwise, put a 0 in the score column.

SCORING: Add the numbers in the score column and enter the sum as the total score. To compute the percentage score, divide the total score by 29 and multiply by 100.

_____ ÷ 29 × 100 = _____

    (total score)   (percentage score)

5. *Policy Clarity*

Section III, Part I   Score

  5. Is there a handbook for residents?....................................Yes No _____

  6. Is there a handbook for staff?..Yes No _____

  7. Is there an orientation program for new residents?..........Yes No _____

  8. Is there an orientation program for new staff?.................Yes No _____

  9. Are there formal staff meetings?.....................................Yes No _____

    9a. Are there formal staff meetings once a
       week or more often?..Yes No _____

    10a. Is there an orientation program for volunteers?
       (n.a. if there are no volunteers.)............................n.a. Yes No _____

Section III, Part V

  6. Is there a newsletter? ....Yes No _____

    6a. Is the newsletter printed once a month
       or more often?..Yes No _____

    7b. Are rules and regulations posted in a
       public location? ....Yes No _____

SCORING: For each yes that has been circled, put a 1 in the score column. For each n.a. that has been circled, write n.a. in the score column. Otherwise, put a 0 in the score column. Add the numbers in the score column and enter the sum as the total score. To obtain the total points possible, subtract the total number of n.a.s from 10. To compute the percentage score, divide the total score by the total points possible and multiply by 100.

$$\underline{\hspace{3cm}} \div \underline{\hspace{4cm}} \times 100 = \underline{\hspace{3.5cm}}$$

     (total score)   (total points possible)   (percentage score)

6. *Provision for Privacy*

Section II   Score

1b. Do at least 50% of the residents have
     a private room or apartment?..Yes No _____

_____ ÷ _____ × 100 = _____%
(total private   (No. of residents)   (% of residents with
rooms and apts.)   private room or apt.)

1f. Do at most two residents share one
     room or dormitory unit?
     (Circle yes if there are apartments only.) ....Yes No _____

1g. Do at least 50% of the residents have
     a private bathroom? ....Yes No _____

_____ ÷ _____ × 100 = _____%
(total private   (No. of residents)   (% of residents
baths and apts.)   with private bath)

1j. Do at most two residents share one bathroom area?
     (Circle yes if there are apartments only.) ....Yes No _____

3b. Do residents have their own individual mailboxes?............Yes No _____

3c. Is there a dresser for each person? ....Yes No _____

3d. Are there locks on all bathroom doors?.............................Yes No _____

Section IV, Part II

14. Are there offices that are closed and private that
     can be used for interviewing residents? ....Yes No _____

STEP 1: For each yes that has been circled, put a 1 in the score column. Otherwise, put a 0 in the score column.

Section III, Part II

What are the rules related to the following behaviors?

	Encouraged Allowed/	Discouraged/ Intolerable	Score
9. Closing the door to one's room............	☐	☐	_____
10. Locking the door to one's room..........	☐	☐	_____

STEP 2: For each encouraged or allowed that has been checked, put a 1 in the score column. Otherwise, put a 0 in the score column.

SCORING: Add the numbers in the score column and enter the sum as the total score. To compute the percentage score, divide the total score by 10 and multiply by 100.

_____ ÷ 10 × 100 = _____

(total score)   (percentage score)

7. Availability of Health Services

Section IV, Part I   Score

Which of the following services are provided by the facility?

1. Regularly scheduled doctor's hours..................................Yes No _____

2. Doctor on call...Yes No _____

3. Regularly scheduled nurse's hours..................................Yes No _____

4. Assistance in using prescribed medications.........................Yes No _____

5. On-site medical clinic ....Yes No _____

6. Physical therapy..Yes No _____

7. Occupational therapy ....Yes No _____

8. Psychotherapy or personal counseling...............................Yes No _____

SCORING: For each yes that has been circled, put a 1 in the score column. Otherwise, put a 0 in the score column. Add the numbers in the score column and enter the sum as the total score. To compute the percentage score, divide the total score by 8 and multiply by 100.

_____ ÷ 8 × 100 = _____

(total score)   (percentage score)

8. *Availability of Daily Living Assistance*

Section IV, Part I   Score

  9. Religious advice or counseling..Yes No _____

10. Legal advice or counseling...Yes No _____

11. Assistance with banking or other financial matters ....Yes No _____

12. Assistance with housekeeping or cleaning ....Yes No _____

14. Assistance with personal care or grooming..........................Yes No _____

15. Barber or beauty service ....Yes No _____

16. Assistance with laundry or linen service ....Yes No _____

17. Assistance with shopping..Yes No _____

18. Providing transportation ....Yes No _____

19. Handling spending money for residents ....Yes No _____

Section IV, Part II

  1. Is breakfast served at least 5 days a week?...........................Yes No _____

  2. Is lunch served at least 5 days a week? ....Yes No _____

  4. Are snacks served in the afternoon or evening?...................Yes No _____

Section IV, Part I

13. Assistance with preparing meals

    OR

Section IV, Part II

  3. Is dinner served at least 5 days a week?...............................Yes No _____

SCORING: For each yes that has been circled, put a 1 in the score column. Otherwise, put a 0 in the score column. Add the numbers in the score column and enter the sum as the total score. To compute the percentage score, divide the total score by 14 and multiply by 100.

$$\underline{\hspace{3cm}} \div 14 \times 100 = \underline{\hspace{3cm}}$$

    (total score)   (percentage score)

9. Availability of Social-Recreational Activities

Section IV, Part III

What is the frequency of each of the following activities?

1 = Very rarely or never
2 = Only a few times a year
3 = Once or twice a month
4 = Once a week or more

	1 or 2	3	4	Score
1. Exercise/physical fitness activity	☐	☐	☐	_____
2. Outside entertainment	☐	☐	☐	_____
3. Discussion groups	☐	☐	☐	_____
4. Reality orientation group	☐	☐	☐	_____
5. Self-help or mutual support group	☐	☐	☐	_____
6. Films or movies	☐	☐	☐	_____
7. Club, social group, or drama or singing groups	☐	☐	☐	_____
8. Classes or lectures	☐	☐	☐	_____
9. Bingo, cards, or other games	☐	☐	☐	_____
10. Parties	☐	☐	☐	_____
11. Religious services	☐	☐	☐	_____
12. Social hour	☐	☐	☐	_____
13. Arts and crafts	☐	☐	☐	_____

SCORING: For each 3 that has been checked, put a 1 in the score column. For each 4 that has been checked, put a 2 in the score column. Otherwise, put a 0 in the score column. Add the numbers in the score column and enter the sum as the total score. To compute the percentage score, divide the total score by 26 and multiply by 100.

_____ ÷ 26 × 100 = _____
   (total score)   (percentage score)

SHELTERED CARE
ENVIRONMENT SCALE (SCES)

Several options are available for scoring the SCES; the option you choose will depend on the number of facilities evaluated, the number of questionnaires completed in each facility, and the personnel and computer time available.

When data are obtained from more than one facility or when large numbers of staff and residents complete the SCES, it is more efficient to computer score the SCES. The scoring key below lists the questions on each subscale and the scoring direction; it can be used to create a computerized scoring system.

The individual's raw score on a dimension is the percentage of questions (out of nine possible) that are answered in the scored direction. The facility's score on a given SCES dimension is the average of all individual scores.

Step-by-step hand-scoring instructions are given under Hand Scoring the SCES.

Scoring Key

Item No.	Cohesion	Conflict	Independence	Self-Disclosure	Organization	Resident Influence	Comfort
1	1Y	2Y	3N	4N	5Y	6N	7Y
2	8Y	9N	10N	11Y	12Y	13Y	14N
3	15N	16Y	17Y	18N	19N	20N	21Y
4	22Y	23N	24Y	25Y	26N	27Y	28N
5	29N	30N	31Y	32N	33Y	34Y	35N
6	36Y	37N	38Y	39Y	40N	41Y	42N
7	43N	44Y	45Y	46Y	47Y	48N	49N
8	50N	51Y	52N	53Y	54N	55N	56Y
9	57Y	58Y	59Y	60N	61N	62Y	63Y

HAND SCORING THE SCES

Hand scoring of the SCES is easier when respondents record their answers directly onto the SCES Answer Sheet (Appendix A). When the SCES is administered to residents in an interview format, the interviewer can record the answers directly onto the answer sheet. If the SCES is administered to staff, it is possible to read questions aloud to the entire group and to have respondents record their answers on this sheet. Use of the answer sheet by respondents should be monitored to ensure accuracy. When respondents have answered the SCES on the questionnaire itself, you can transfer answers from the forms to answer sheets to facilitate hand scoring with the scoring template.

STEP 1: Discard questionnaires with more than 10 unanswered questions.

STEP 2: If respondents have marked on the questionnaire rather than on the answer sheet, transfer answers to the answer sheet (Appendix A). A separate answer sheet should be used for each respondent.

STEP 3: Cut out the boxes marked with an "X" on the scoring template. The columns on the template are labeled with the SCES subscale names. Each of the seven columns contains all the items used in scoring one SCES subscale (e.g., Items 1, 8, 15, 22, 29, 36, 43, 50, and 57 are on the Cohesion subscale; Items 2, 9, 16, 23, 30, 37, 44, 51, and 58 are on the Conflict subscale, etc.).

STEP 4: Align the scoring template over an answer sheet. Obtain the raw score for Cohesion by counting the number of responses appearing in the windows of column 1.

STEP 5: Divide the raw score by 9 (the total points possible on each subscale and multiply by 100). This is the individual's percentage score for Cohesion.

STEP 6: Repeat Steps 4 and 5 for each of the subscales, recording the respondent's percentage scores. Score each person's SCES in this way, keeping resident and staff groups separate.

STEP 7: To calculate facility SCES scores, average the individual percentage scores for each of the subscales. You should end up with seven facility means (one for each subscale) for the resident group and seven for the staff group.

	Cohesion	Conflict	Independence	Self-Disclosure	Organization	Resident Influence	Comfort	
	COL 1	COL 2	COL 3	COL 4	COL 5	COL 6	COL 7	
	Item 1	Item 2	Item 3	Item 4	Item 5	Item 6	Item 7	
Yes	X	X			X		X	Yes
No			X	X		X		No
	Item 8	Item 9	Item 10	Item 11	Item 12	Item 13	Item 14	
Yes	X			X	X	X		Yes
No		X	X				X	No
	Item 15	Item 16	Item 17	Item 18	Item 19	Item 20	Item 21	
Yes		X	X				X	Yes
No	X			X	X	X		No
	Item 22	Item 23	Item 24	Item 25	Item 26	Item 27	Item 28	
Yes	X		X	X		X		Yes
No		X			X		X	No
	Item 29	Item 30	Item 31	Item 32	Item 33	Item 34	Item 35	
Yes			X		X	X		Yes
No	X	X		X			X	No
	Item 36	Item 37	Item 38	Item 39	Item 40	Item 41	Item 42	
Yes	X		X	X		X		Yes
No		X			X		X	No
	Item 43	Item 44	Item 45	Item 46	Item 47	Item 48	Item 49	
Yes		X	X	X	X			Yes
No	X					X	X	No
	Item 50	Item 51	Item 52	Item 53	Item 54	Item 55	Item 56	
Yes		X		X			X	Yes
No	X		X		X	X		No
	Item 57	Item 58	Item 59	Item 60	Item 61	Item 62	Item 63	
Yes	X	X	X			X	X	Yes
No				X	X			No

RATING SCALE

If several raters have rated a facility, average their ratings together before completing hand scoring. Compute a single rating for each Rating Scale item by averaging the ratings for the four areas (lounge, dining room, bedrooms, and hallways). If the facility lacks a particular area, such as hallways, average ratings on the applicable areas. Transfer the information from the Rating Scale (section and item number are indicated for each question).

1. Physical Attractiveness

Section I   Score

  1. As a neighborhood for living, how does the area around this site look? ...._____

  2. How attractive are the site grounds? ...._____

  3. How attractive are the site buildings? ...._____

Section II, Part I

  1. Noise level (average rating) ...._____

  2. Odors (average rating).._____

  3. Level of illumination (average rating)..._____

  4. Cleanliness of walls and floors (average rating)............................_____

  5. Condition of walls and floors (average rating) ...._____

  6. Condition of furniture (average rating)..._____

SCORING: Add the numbers in the score column and enter the sum as the total score. To obtain the total points possible, subtract the total number of missing ratings from 9 and multiply by 3 (the maximum possible rating). To compute the percentage score, divide the total score by the total points possible and multiply by 100.

_____ ÷ _____ × 100 = _____

(total score)   (total points possible)   (percentage score)

2. *Environmental Diversity*

Section II, Part I   Score

  7. Window areas (average rating) ...._____

  8. View from windows—interest (average rating) ...._____

Section II, Part II

  9. Variation in design of residents' rooms (apartments) ...._____

10. Personalization of residents' rooms (apartments)........................._____

11. Distinctiveness of all living spaces..._____

SCORING: Add the numbers in the score column and enter the sum as the total score. To obtain the total points possible, subtract the total number of missing ratings from 5 and multiply by 3 (the maximum possible rating). To compute the percentage score, divide the total score by the total points possible and multiply by 100.

$$\underline{\hspace{2cm}} \div \underline{\hspace{3cm}} \times 100 = \underline{\hspace{3cm}}$$

    (total score)   (total points possible)   (percentage score)

3. *Resident Functioning*

Section III   Score

  1. Personal grooming..._____

  2. Condition of clothing..._____

  3. Interaction of residents..._____

  4. Brief verbal exchanges..._____

  5. General amount of activity.._____

SCORING: Add the numbers in the score column and enter the sum as the total score. To obtain the total points possible, subtract the total number of missing ratings from 5 and multiply by 3 (the maximum possible rating). To compute the percentage score, divide the total score by the total points possible and multiply by 100.

$$\underline{\hspace{2cm}} \div \underline{\hspace{3cm}} \times 100 = \underline{\hspace{3cm}}$$

    (total score)   (total points possible)   (percentage score)

4. Staff Functioning

Section IV   Score

1. Quality of interaction .... _____
2. Physical contact with residents .... _____
3. Organization.. _____
4. Availability of staff to residents .... _____
5. Staff conflict .... _____

**SCORING: Add the numbers in the score column and enter the sum as the total
score. To obtain the total points possible, subtract the total number of missing
ratings from 5 and multiply by 3 (the maximum possible rating). To compute the
percentage score, divide the total score by the total points possible and multiply
by 100.**

$$\underline{\hspace{2cm}} \div \underline{\hspace{3cm}} \times 100 = \underline{\hspace{3cm}}$$

(total score)   (total points possible)   (percentage score)

Appendix C:
Standard Score
Conversion Tables

CALCULATION OF STANDARD SCORES

To convert a subscale percentage score (X) to a standard score (z), we used the mean ($\overline{X}$) and standard deviation (SD) of the normative sample in the following formula: $z = 10[(X - \overline{X}) \div SD] + 50$.

Table C.1 shows the standard score conversion table for the Resident and Staff Information Form (RESIF). Percentage scores are in the first column; standard scores for three subscales are in the other columns. The table includes standard scores for the total sample and three subsamples. Using the total sample, a percentage score of 55 on Resident Social Resources equals a standard score of 60, which is 1 SD above the mean. For nursing homes, a percentage score of 55 on Resident Social Resources equals a standard score of 65.

The tables do not include every possible percentage score. To convert a percentage score that is not shown in the table, use interpolation. For example, take a percentage score of 47 on Resident Social Resources. Because 47 is two fifths of the way between 45 and 50, which are shown in the table, its standard score is two fifths of the way between the standard scores for 45 and for 50, which are 54 and 57, respectively. Thus, a percentage score of 57 equals a standard score of 55 on Resident Social Resources.

TABLE C.1 RESIF Percentage Score to Standard Score Conversion Table

Percent-age Score	Resident Social Resources				Resident Heterogeneity				Resident Functional Abilities			
	Total Sample	NH	RC	APT	Total Sample	NH	RC	APT	Total Sample	NH	RC	APT
100	86	94	79	86	78	79	82	74	64	100	65	65
95	83	91	77	83	76	77	79	72	63	96	62	55
90	80	88	74	80	73	74	77	70	61	92	58	45
85	77	85	71	76	71	72	75	68	59	88	55	36
80	74	81	68	73	69	69	72	66	57	84	52	26
75	71	78	66	70	66	67	70	64	55	80	48	16
70	68	75	63	66	64	64	67	62	53	76	45	6
65	66	72	60	63	62	62	65	60	52	72	41	—
60	63	68	58	60	59	59	63	58	50	68	38	—
55	60	65	55	56	57	56	60	56	48	64	35	—
50	57	62	52	53	55	54	58	53	46	60	31	—
45	54	58	50	50	52	51	55	51	44	56	28	—
40	51	55	47	46	50	49	53	49	42	52	24	—
35	48	52	44	43	48	46	50	47	41	48	21	—
30	45	49	42	39	45	44	48	45	39	44	17	—
25	42	45	39	36	43	41	46	43	37	40	14	—
20	39	42	36	33	41	39	43	41	35	36	11	—
15	36	39	34	29	38	36	41	39	33	32	7	—
10	34	36	31	26	36	34	38	37	31	28	4	—
5	31	32	28	23	33	31	36	35	30	24	0	—
0	28	29	25	19	31	29	34	33	28	20	—	—

NOTE: NH = nursing home; RC = residential care; APT = apartment.

TABLE C.1 *Continued*

Percent-age Score	Resident Activity Level				Resident Activities in the Community				Staff Resources			
	Total Sample	NH	RC	APTS	Total Sample	NH	RC	APTS	Total Sample	NH	RC	APT
100	94	—	99	97	89	—	95	81	77	78	81	98
95	90	—	95	93	87	—	92	79	74	75	78	94
90	87	—	90	88	84	—	89	76	72	72	76	91
85	84	—	86	83	81	—	86	73	69	68	73	88
80	80	—	82	79	79	99	83	70	67	65	71	84
75	77	97	78	74	76	95	80	68	64	61	68	81
70	74	92	74	69	74	91	76	65	62	58	66	77
65	70	87	69	64	71	87	73	62	59	54	63	74
60	67	82	65	60	68	84	70	59	56	51	60	70
55	63	78	61	55	66	80	67	57	54	48	58	67
50	60	73	57	50	63	76	64	54	51	44	55	63
45	57	68	53	46	61	72	61	51	49	41	53	60
40	53	63	48	41	58	69	58	48	46	37	50	56
35	50	59	44	36	55	65	55	46	44	34	47	53
30	47	54	40	31	53	61	52	43	41	30	45	50
25	43	49	36	27	50	57	48	40	39	27	42	46
20	40	44	32	22	47	54	45	37	36	24	40	43
15	37	40	27	17	45	50	42	35	34	20	37	39
10	33	35	23	13	42	46	39	32	31	17	35	36
5	30	30	19	8	40	42	36	29	29	13	32	32
0	27	25	15	3	37	39	33	26	26	10	29	29

NOTE: NH = nursing home; RC = residential care; APT = apartment.

TABLE C.2 PAF Form R Percentage Score to Standard Score Conversion Table

Percent-age Score	Community Accessibility				Physical Amenities				Social-Recreational Aids			
	Total Sample	NH	RC	APT	Total Sample	NH	RC	APT	Total Sample	NH	RC	APT
100	71	73	70	70	77	78	74	77	75	77	72	74
95	69	71	68	68	73	74	71	73	71	73	69	71
90	67	69	66	65	69	70	68	70	68	70	66	68
85	65	67	64	63	66	66	65	66	65	66	63	64
80	63	65	62	60	62	62	61	62	61	62	60	61
75	61	63	60	58	58	58	58	59	58	59	57	58
70	59	61	58	55	54	54	55	55	55	55	54	55
65	56	59	56	53	51	50	52	51	51	51	51	52
60	54	57	54	50	47	46	49	48	48	47	48	48
55	52	55	52	48	43	42	45	44	44	44	45	45
50	50	53	50	45	40	38	42	41	41	40	42	42
45	48	51	48	43	36	33	39	37	38	36	39	39
40	46	49	46	40	32	29	36	33	34	33	36	36
35	44	47	44	38	29	25	33	30	31	29	33	32
30	42	45	42	35	25	21	29	26	28	25	30	29
25	40	43	40	33	21	17	26	22	24	21	27	26
20	38	41	38	30	17	13	23	19	21	18	24	23
15	36	39	36	27	14	9	20	15	17	14	21	20
10	34	37	34	25	10	5	17	12	14	10	18	16
5	32	35	32	22	6	1	13	8	11	7	15	13
0	30	33	30	20	3	—	10	4	7	3	12	10

NOTE: NH = nursing home; RC = residential care; APT = apartment.

TABLE C.2 *Continued*

Percent-age Score	Total Sample	Prosthetic Aids NH	RC	APT	Total Sample	Orientational Aids NH	RC	APT	Total Sample	Safety Features NH	RC	APT
100	70	76	77	94	85	86	86	86	69	71	71	67
95	67	70	74	90	81	82	83	82	66	67	68	64
90	64	64	71	85	78	79	80	78	63	64	65	61
85	61	59	68	80	74	75	77	75	60	61	62	58
80	58	53	66	76	71	71	74	71	57	57	59	55
75	56	47	63	71	67	67	70	67	54	54	57	52
70	53	41	60	66	64	63	67	64	51	51	54	49
65	50	36	57	62	60	59	64	60	48	47	51	46
60	47	30	54	57	57	55	61	57	45	44	48	44
55	44	24	52	52	53	51	58	53	42	40	45	41
50	41	19	49	48	50	48	54	49	39	37	43	38
45	38	13	46	43	46	44	51	46	36	34	40	35
40	35	7	43	38	43	40	48	42	33	30	37	32
35	32	1	41	34	39	36	45	38	30	27	34	29
30	30	—	38	29	36	32	41	35	27	24	31	26
25	27	—	35	24	32	28	38	31	24	20	29	23
20	24	—	32	20	29	24	35	28	21	17	26	20
15	21	—	29	15	25	20	32	24	18	14	23	17
10	18	—	27	10	22	17	29	20	14	10	20	14
5	15	—	24	6	18	13	25	17	11	7	17	11
0	12	—	21	1	15	9	22	13	8	4	15	8

NOTE: NH = nursing home; RC = residential care; APT = apartment.

TABLE C.2 *Continued*

Percent- age Score		Staff Facilities				Space Availability		
	Total Sample	NH	RC	APT	Total Sample	NH	RC	APT
100	67	68	67	75	72	75	69	74
95	65	66	65	73	70	73	66	71
90	63	63	63	71	68	71	64	69
85	61	60	62	68	66	68	61	66
80	59	57	60	66	63	66	59	64
75	57	54	59	63	61	64	56	62
70	55	52	57	61	59	61	54	59
65	53	49	55	59	56	59	51	57
60	51	46	54	56	54	57	49	54
55	49	43	52	54	52	54	46	52
50	47	41	51	52	50	52	44	49
45	45	38	49	49	47	50	41	47
40	43	35	47	47	45	48	39	44
35	41	32	46	45	43	45	36	42
30	39	29	44	42	41	43	34	40
25	37	27	42	40	38	41	31	37
20	35	24	41	38	36	38	29	35
15	33	21	39	35	34	36	26	32
10	31	18	38	33	31	34	24	30
5	28	15	36	30	29	31	21	27
0	26	13	34	28	27	29	19	25

NOTE: NH = nursing home; RC = residential care; APT = apartment.

TABLE C.3   POLIF Percentage Score to Standard Score Conversion Table

Percent-age Score	Total Sample	Expectations for Functioning NH	RC	APT	Total Sample	Acceptance of Problem Behavior NH	RC	APT	Total Sample	Policy Choice NH	RC	APT
100	69	—	74	63	75	73	77	80	68	83	72	67
95	68	—	72	60	72	71	74	77	66	80	70	62
90	66	—	70	57	70	68	72	74	64	77	68	56
85	65	98	68	54	68	66	70	71	62	74	65	51
80	63	94	66	51	65	64	68	68	60	71	63	46
75	62	91	64	48	63	62	66	65	58	68	61	40
70	60	88	62	45	61	60	63	62	56	66	59	35
65	59	85	60	42	59	58	61	59	54	63	56	29
60	57	82	58	39	56	55	59	56	52	60	54	24
55	56	78	55	36	54	53	57	53	50	57	52	18
50	54	75	53	33	52	51	55	50	48	54	50	13
45	53	72	51	30	49	49	52	47	46	51	48	8
40	51	69	49	27	47	47	50	44	44	48	45	2
35	50	66	47	24	45	45	48	41	42	45	43	—
30	49	62	45	21	43	43	46	38	40	42	41	—
25	47	59	43	18	40	40	44	35	37	40	39	—
20	46	56	41	15	38	38	42	32	35	37	36	—
15	44	53	39	12	36	36	39	29	33	34	34	—
10	43	50	37	9	34	34	37	26	31	31	32	—
5	41	46	35	6	31	32	35	23	29	28	30	—
0	40	43	32	2	29	30	33	20	27	25	27	—

NOTE: NH = nursing home; RC = residential care; APT = apartment.

TABLE C.3 *Continued*

Percent- age Score	Resident Control				Policy Clarity				Provision for Privacy			
	Total Sample	NH	RC	APTS	Total Sample	NH	RC	APTS	Total Sample	NH	RC	APT
100	83	92	80	80	67	70	67	68	65	98	66	60
95	80	89	78	77	65	66	66	66	64	95	64	52
90	78	86	76	74	63	63	64	64	62	91	63	45
85	75	83	73	71	60	60	62	62	60	87	61	38
80	73	80	71	68	58	57	60	60	59	84	59	31
75	70	77	69	65	56	54	58	57	57	80	57	23
70	67	74	66	62	53	51	56	55	55	76	55	16
65	65	71	64	59	51	48	54	53	54	73	53	9
60	62	68	62	56	49	44	52	51	52	69	52	2
55	60	65	59	54	46	41	50	49	50	65	50	—
50	57	62	57	51	44	38	48	46	48	61	48	—
45	54	59	54	48	42	35	46	44	47	58	46	—
40	52	56	52	45	39	32	44	42	45	54	44	—
35	49	53	50	42	37	29	42	40	43	50	42	—
30	47	50	47	39	34	26	40	38	42	47	40	—
25	44	47	45	36	32	22	38	35	40	43	39	—
20	41	43	43	33	30	19	36	33	38	39	37	—
15	39	40	40	30	27	16	34	31	37	36	35	—
10	36	37	38	27	25	13	33	29	35	32	33	—
5	34	34	36	24	23	10	31	27	33	28	31	—
0	31	31	33	21	20	7	29	24	32	25	29	—

NOTE: NH = nursing home; RC = residential care; APT = apartment.

TABLE C.3 *Continued*

Percent-age Score	Total Sample	Availability of Health Services			Total Sample	Availability of Daily Living Assistance			Total Sample	Availability of Social-Recreational Activities		
		NH	RC	APT		NH	RC	APT		NH	RC	APT
100	69	75	74	—	61	64	67	85	67	68	68	77
95	68	72	72	—	59	59	63	83	65	65	66	75
90	66	68	70	98	57	53	60	80	63	61	64	72
85	64	65	68	95	56	48	56	77	60	58	62	69
80	62	61	66	91	54	43	53	75	58	55	60	67
75	60	57	64	88	52	37	49	72	56	52	58	64
70	59	54	62	85	50	32	46	70	54	48	56	62
65	57	50	60	82	48	26	42	67	51	45	54	59
60	55	47	58	79	46	21	39	65	49	42	52	57
55	53	43	56	76	44	16	35	62	47	38	51	54
50	51	39	54	73	42	10	31	59	45	35	49	51
45	50	36	52	70	41	5	28	57	43	32	47	49
40	48	32	50	67	39	—	24	54	40	29	45	46
35	46	29	48	63	37	—	21	52	38	25	43	44
30	44	25	46	60	35	—	17	49	36	22	41	41
25	42	22	44	57	33	—	14	46	34	19	39	38
20	41	18	42	54	31	—	10	44	31	16	37	36
15	39	14	40	51	29	—	7	41	29	12	35	33
10	37	11	38	48	27	—	3	39	27	9	33	31
5	35	7	36	45	26	—	—	36	25	6	32	28
0	33	4	34	42	24	—	—	34	22	2	30	25

NOTE: NH = nursing home; RC = residential care; APT = apartment.

TABLE C.4 SCES Percentage Score to Standard Score Conversion Table (Based on Resident Samples)

Percent- age Score	Cohesion				Conflict				Independence			
	Total Sample	NH	RC	APT	Total Sample	NH	RC	APT	Total Sample	NH	RC	APT
100	80	83	77	78	100	100	—	—	90	99	89	91
95	76	79	73	74	97	96	99	—	86	95	85	86
90	72	74	69	70	93	92	96	99	82	90	81	81
85	68	70	66	66	89	88	92	95	78	85	78	76
80	64	66	62	62	85	84	88	91	74	81	74	71
75	60	61	58	58	82	80	84	87	70	76	70	66
70	56	57	54	54	78	76	81	83	66	71	67	60
65	51	53	50	50	74	72	77	79	62	67	63	55
60	47	49	47	46	70	68	73	75	58	62	59	50
55	43	44	43	42	67	64	69	71	54	57	56	45
50	39	40	39	38	63	61	66	67	50	53	52	40
45	35	36	35	34	59	57	62	63	45	48	48	35
40	31	31	31	30	55	53	58	59	41	43	44	29
35	27	27	27	26	52	49	55	55	37	39	41	24
30	23	23	24	22	48	45	51	51	33	34	37	19
25	19	18	20	18	44	41	47	47	29	29	33	14
20	15	14	16	15	40	37	43	43	25	25	30	9
15	10	10	12	11	37	33	40	39	21	20	26	4
10	6	5	8	7	33	29	36	35	17	15	22	—
5	2	1	5	3	29	25	32	31	13	11	19	—
0	—	—	1	—	25	21	28	27	9	6	15	—

NOTE: NH = nursing home; RC = residential care; APT = apartment.

TABLE C.4 *Continued*

Percent-age Score	Self-Disclosure				Organization				Resident Influence			
	Total Sample	NH	RC	APT	Total Sample	NH	RC	APT	Total Sample	NH	RC	APT
100	—	—	—	—	78	84	75	75	—	—	99	—
95	—	—	—	—	73	79	70	70	—	98	94	—
90	—	—	—	—	69	75	66	65	96	93	90	—
85	—	—	96	—	64	70	61	61	91	88	85	—
80	97	99	91	—	60	65	57	56	86	84	81	100
75	92	93	87	100	56	60	52	52	81	79	77	93
70	87	88	82	93	51	55	48	47	76	75	72	86
65	81	83	78	86	47	50	43	42	71	70	68	79
60	76	77	73	79	42	46	39	38	66	65	63	72
55	71	72	68	73	38	41	34	33	61	61	59	65
50	65	67	64	66	34	36	30	28	56	56	54	58
45	60	61	59	59	29	31	25	24	51	52	50	51
40	55	56	55	52	25	26	21	19	46	47	46	44
35	49	51	50	46	21	22	16	15	41	42	41	37
30	44	45	46	39	16	17	12	10	36	38	37	30
25	39	40	41	32	12	12	7	5	31	33	32	23
20	33	35	36	25	7	7	3	1	26	29	28	16
15	28	29	32	19	3	2	—	—	21	24	23	9
10	23	24	27	12	—	—	—	—	16	20	19	2
5	17	19	23	5	—	—	—	—	11	15	15	—
0	12	13	18	—	—	—	—	—	7	10	10	—

NOTE: NH = nursing home; RC = residential care; APT = apartment.

TABLE C.4 *Continued*

Percen-tage Score	Total Sample	Physical Comfort		
		NH	RC	APT
100	67	74	64	65
95	62	69	59	59
90	58	64	54	53
85	54	59	50	47
80	49	54	45	41
75	45	50	41	35
70	40	45	36	29
65	36	40	32	23
60	32	35	27	17
55	27	30	22	10
50	23	25	18	4
45	19	20	13	—
40	14	16	9	—
35	10	11	4	—
30	5	6	—	—
25	1	1	—	—
20	—	—	—	—
15	—	—	—	—
10	—	—	—	—
5	—	—	—	—
0	—	—	—	—

NOTE: NH = nursing home; RC = residential care; APT = apartment.

TABLE C.5 SCES Percentage Score to Standard Score Conversion Table
(Based on Staff Samples)

Percent- age Score	Cohesion				Conflict				Independence			
	Total Sample	NH	RC	APT	Total Sample	NH	RC	APT	Total Sample	NH	RC	APT
100	73	78	68	69	76	80	77	79	80	98	81	70
95	68	74	65	65	73	76	74	76	77	93	77	67
90	64	69	61	61	70	72	71	73	73	88	74	64
85	60	64	58	58	67	68	69	70	70	83	70	61
80	56	60	54	54	64	64	66	67	66	77	67	57
75	52	55	50	50	61	59	64	65	62	72	64	54
70	48	51	47	46	58	55	61	62	59	67	60	51
65	44	46	43	42	55	51	58	59	55	62	57	48
60	40	41	40	38	52	47	56	56	52	56	53	45
55	36	37	36	34	49	43	53	53	48	51	50	41
50	32	32	32	30	46	39	50	50	44	46	47	38
45	28	27	29	27	43	35	48	47	41	41	43	35
40	24	23	25	23	40	30	45	45	37	36	40	32
35	20	18	22	19	37	26	43	42	34	30	36	29
30	16	14	18	15	34	22	40	39	30	25	33	25
25	12	9	14	11	31	18	37	36	26	20	30	22
20	8	4	11	7	28	14	35	33	23	15	26	19
15	4	0	7	3	25	10	32	30	19	10	23	16
10	—	—	4	—	22	6	30	27	16	4	19	13
5	—	—	—	—	19	2	27	25	12	—	16	9
0	—	—	—	—	16	—	24	22	8	—	13	6

NOTE: NH = nursing home; RC = residential care; APT = apartment.

TABLE C.5 *Continued*

Percent- age Score	Self-Disclosure Total Sample	NH	RC	APT	Organization Total Sample	NH	RC	APT	Resident Influence Total Sample	NH	RC	APT
100	80	87	76	79	74	81	70	70	83	93	75	80
95	76	82	73	75	70	77	66	67	79	87	71	76
90	73	77	69	72	67	73	63	63	75	82	68	72
85	69	72	66	68	63	69	59	60	70	77	65	69
80	65	67	63	65	60	65	55	56	66	71	62	65
75	61	62	60	62	56	61	51	52	62	66	59	61
70	57	57	56	58	53	57	48	49	58	60	56	57
65	53	52	53	55	49	53	44	45	54	55	53	54
60	49	47	50	51	45	49	40	42	50	50	50	50
55	45	42	47	48	42	45	37	38	46	44	47	46
50	41	37	44	45	38	41	33	34	41	39	44	43
45	37	32	40	41	35	37	29	31	37	34	40	39
40	34	27	37	38	31	33	26	27	33	28	37	35
35	30	22	34	35	28	29	22	24	29	23	34	31
30	26	17	31	31	24	25	18	20	25	17	31	28
25	22	12	27	28	21	21	15	16	21	12	28	24
20	18	7	24	24	17	17	11	13	17	7	25	20
15	14	2	21	21	14	13	7	9	13	1	22	16
10	10	—	18	18	10	9	4	6	8	—	19	13
5	6	—	14	14	6	5	1	2	4	—	16	9
0	2	—	11	11	3	1	—	—	0	—	12	5

NOTE: NH = nursing home; RC = residential care; APT = apartment.

TABLE C.5 *Continued*

Percentage Score	Total Sample	Physical Comfort		
		NH	RC	APT
100	65	76	62	62
95	62	72	58	57
90	59	68	53	53
85	55	64	49	48
80	52	60	45	43
75	49	56	40	39
70	45	52	36	34
65	42	48	32	29
60	39	44	28	25
55	36	40	23	20
50	32	36	19	16
45	29	31	15	11
40	26	27	11	6
35	22	23	6	2
30	19	19	2	—
25	16	15	—	—
20	12	11	—	—
15	9	7	—	—
10	6	3	—	—
5	2	—	—	—
0	—	—	—	—

NOTE: NH = nursing home; RC = residential care; APT = apartment.

TABLE C.6 Rating Scale Percentage Score to Standard Score Conversion Table

Percentage Score	Physical Attractiveness				Environmental Diversity				Resident Functioning			
	Total Sample	NH	RC	APT	Total Sample	NH	RC	APT	Total Sample	NH	RC	APT
100	73	79	70	68	72	79	72	73	65	72	65	60
95	69	75	67	65	69	76	70	68	63	69	63	56
90	66	70	64	62	67	73	67	64	60	67	60	53
85	62	66	60	59	64	70	64	60	58	64	58	50
80	59	62	57	56	61	67	61	55	56	61	55	46
75	55	58	54	53	58	64	58	51	53	58	53	43
70	52	53	51	50	56	61	55	46	51	56	51	40
65	48	49	48	47	53	58	52	42	48	53	48	37
60	44	45	44	43	50	55	49	37	46	50	46	33
55	41	40	41	40	47	52	47	33	44	48	43	30
50	37	36	38	37	45	49	44	28	41	45	41	27
45	34	32	35	34	42	46	41	24	39	42	39	24
40	30	28	32	31	39	43	38	19	37	40	36	20
35	26	23	28	28	36	40	35	15	34	37	34	17
30	23	19	25	25	34	37	32	10	32	34	31	14
25	19	15	22	22	31	34	29	6	30	31	29	11
20	16	11	19	18	28	31	26	—	27	29	26	7
15	12	6	16	15	25	28	24	—	25	26	24	4
10	8	2	13	12	22	25	21	—	23	23	22	1
5	5	—	9	9	20	22	18	—	20	21	19	—
0	1	—	6	6	17	19	15	—	18	18	17	—

NOTE: NH, nursing home; RC, residential care; APT, apartment.

TABLE C.6 *Continued*

Percentage Score	Total Sample	Staff Functioning		
		NH	RC	APT
100	68	66	70	75
95	65	63	67	72
90	63	60	64	69
85	60	57	61	66
80	57	54	58	63
75	54	51	55	60
70	51	48	52	56
65	48	46	49	53
60	46	43	46	50
55	43	40	43	47
50	40	37	40	44
45	37	34	37	41
40	34	31	34	38
35	31	28	31	35
30	29	25	28	32
25	26	22	26	29
20	23	19	23	26
15	20	17	20	23
10	17	14	17	20
5	15	11	14	17
0	12	8	11	14

NOTE: NH, nursing home; RC, residential care; APT, apartment.

Appendix D: Physical and Architectural Features (PAF) Form I,
Policy and Program Information (POLIF) Form I,
Sheltered Care Environment Scale (SCES) Form I,
Scoring Directions, and Norms on a 4-Point Scale

PHYSICAL AND ARCHITECTURAL
FEATURES CHECKLIST FORM I

In the next few years, new types of housing will be designed for older adults. We want to know what you think is most important in an *ideal* group living setting for older adults. Please answer the questions to describe the *best possible* living environment.

Many older adults find that they can no longer live alone in their own home or apartment. This may happen because they are in poor health, because their husband or wife has died, because it has become too expensive to keep up a house, or because of some combination of these factors. In such a situation, one alternative is to move to a group living setting in which there are rooms or apartments and in which meals are provided.

If the above statement described your situation, what would the *best possible* place for you be like? We would like you to tell us whether each feature of the physical environment would be part of an *ideal* setting for you.

> *Not Important*—this means that a feature would be not important in your ideal setting.
>
> *Desirable*—this means that a feature would be desirable in your ideal setting.
>
> *Very Important*—this means that a feature would be very important in your ideal setting.
>
> *Essential*—this means that a feature would be essential in your ideal setting.

Place an "X" in the box for the answer that best describes your *ideal* setting. Please be sure to answer every question. Thank you for your help.

Your name (optional) _____ Date _____

Your age _____   Male ☐   Female ☐

Where do you live now? _____

How long have you lived there? _____

Part I: Neighborhood Context

	Not Important	Desirable	Very Important	Essential
	1	2	3	4

1. Should the following community resources be located within easy walking *walking* distance of the facility (1/4 mile)?

	Not Important	Desirable	Very Important	Essential
1a. Grocery store	☐	☐	☐	☐ 1
1b. Drugstore	☐	☐	☐	☐
1c. Senior citizens center	☐	☐	☐	☐
1d. Movie theater	☐	☐	☐	☐
1e. Church or synagogue	☐	☐	☐	☐ 5
1f. Public library	☐	☐	☐	☐
1g. Bank	☐	☐	☐	☐
1h. Hospital	☐	☐	☐	☐
1i. Doctor's office	☐	☐	☐	☐
1j. Dentist's office	☐	☐	☐	☐ 10
1k. Post office	☐	☐	☐	☐
1l. Park	☐	☐	☐	☐

2. Should the city or town within which this facility is located have a public transportation system? ☐ ☐ ☐ ☐

3. Should a public transportation stop be within easy walking distance (1/4 mile)? ☐ ☐ ☐ ☐

3a. If so, should it have benches? ☐ ☐ ☐ ☐

4. Should there be lights in the surrounding streets? ☐ ☐ ☐ ☐ 16

Part II: Exterior of Building

	Not Important	Desirable	Very Important	Essential
	1	2	3	4

1. Should the main entrance be sheltered from sun and rain? ☐ ☐ ☐ ☐ 17

2. Should the area outside the building be well lighted? ☐ ☐ ☐ ☐

	Not Important	Desirable	Very Important	Essential
	1	2	3	4
3. Should the outside walk and entrance be visible				
3a. from seating spaces in the lobby or a ground floor social space?	☐	☐	☐	☐
3b. from the office or station of an employee?	☐	☐	☐	☐ 20
4. Should there be outside seating in the front of the building?	☐	☐	☐	☐
4a. For safety, should it be visible from the entrance lobby or a ground floor social space?	☐	☐	☐	☐
4b. For safety, should it be visible from the office or station of an employee?	☐	☐	☐	☐
4c. Should it be protected from the weather?	☐	☐	☐	☐
4d. Should it provide a view of pedestrians and other activity?	☐	☐	☐	☐ 25
5. Should there be a patio or open courtyard?	☐	☐	☐	☐
6. Consider the outside of the building:				
6a. Should tables be available?	☐	☐	☐	☐
6b. Should umbrella tables be available?	☐	☐	☐	☐
6c. Should the outdoor furniture be in good condition?	☐	☐	☐	☐
6d. Should there be a covered area that is rainproof?	☐	☐	☐	☐ 30
6e. Should there be an area with a sunscreen (not necessarily rainproof) or protection from the sun (e.g., trees)?	☐	☐	☐	☐ 31
6f. Should there be a barbecue?	☐	☐	☐	☐
6g. Should there be a shuffleboard game area?	☐	☐	☐	☐
7. Should there be a garden area for resident use?	☐	☐	☐	☐
8. Should there be a lawn?	☐	☐	☐	☐ 35

	Not Important	Desirable	Very Important	Essential
	1	2	3	4
9. Should there be reserved parking for handicapped people?	☐	☐	☐	☐
10. Should there be parking for staff?	☐	☐	☐	☐
11. Should there be parking for visitors?	☐	☐	☐	☐

Part III: Lobby and Entrance Area

	Not Important	Desirable	Very Important	Essential
1. Should one be able to enter the building from the street without having to use any stairs?	☐	☐	☐	☐
2. For safety, should entry from outside be limited to at most one unlocked door?	☐	☐	☐	☐ 40
3. Should there be a bell or call system outside?	☐	☐	☐	☐
4. Should written instructions be posted outside that explain how to get in if the front door is locked?	☐	☐	☐	☐
5. Should the front door open automatically?	☐	☐	☐	☐
6. Should the front door swing closed by itself?	☐	☐	☐	☐
7. Should the front door be wide enough for a wheelchair?	☐	☐	☐	☐ 45
8. For safety, should there be an individual who usually monitors the entrance to the building?	☐	☐	☐	☐ 46
9. Should there be a reception area or reception desk?	☐	☐	☐	☐
10. Should there be a place for visitors to sign in?	☐	☐	☐	☐
11. Should there be seating in the lobby?	☐	☐	☐	☐
12. Should there be a comfortably furnished lounge near the entrance?	☐	☐	☐	☐ 50
13. Should one be able to see into the lobby or entrance area from a community room or other ground floor social space?	☐	☐	☐	☐
14. Should there be at least one large clock in the lobby or entrance area?	☐	☐	☐	☐

Part IV: Lounge and Community Room Areas

	Not Important	Desirable	Very Important	Essential
	1	2	3	4
1. Should the hallways be wide enough for two wheelchairs to pass each other?	☐	☐	☐	☐
2. Should the hallways be uncrowded and free of obstructions?	☐	☐	☐	☐
3. Should there be handrails in the halls?	☐	☐	☐	☐ 55
4. Should the halls be decorated (e.g., with pictures or plants)?	☐	☐	☐	☐
5. Should there be drinking fountains?	☐	☐	☐	☐
5a. Should they be accessible to wheelchair residents?	☐	☐	☐	☐
5b. Should there be at least one drinking fountain on each floor of the building?	☐	☐	☐	☐ 59
6. Should there be public telephones?	☐	☐	☐	☐ 1
6a. Should there be a writing surface by the telephone?	☐	☐	☐	☐
6b. Should at least one public phone be accessible to wheelchair residents?	☐	☐	☐	☐
6c. Should at least one phone have a loudness control in the receiver for people who are hard of hearing?	☐	☐	☐	☐
6d. Should there be at least one public phone on each floor of the building?	☐	☐	☐	☐ 5
7. Should there be smoke detection devices in the halls?	☐	☐	☐	☐
8. Should a resident be able to go anywhere in the building without having to climb *any* steps?	☐	☐	☐	☐
9. Should all stairs be well lighted?	☐	☐	☐	☐
10. Should there be nonskid surfaces on stairs and ramps?	☐	☐	☐	☐
11. Should each corridor or floor be color coded or numbered?	☐	☐	☐	☐ 10
12. Should residents' names be on or next to their doors?	☐	☐	☐	☐
13. Should it be easy for new residents to find their way around the building?	☐	☐	☐	☐

Part V: Lounge and Community Room Areas

	Not Important	Desirable	Very Important	Essential
	1	2	3	4
1. Should there be at least two rooms for resident activities (such as visiting, playing cards, and social activities)?	☐	☐	☐	☐
2. Should at least one of these rooms be near an entrance or traveled hallway?	☐	☐	☐	☐ 14
3. Should there be writing desks or tables?	☐	☐	☐	☐ 15
4. Should there be small tables for several people to sit and talk or play games?	☐	☐	☐	☐
5. Should reading material be available on tables or shelves?	☐	☐	☐	☐
6. Should there be table lamps in the lounges?	☐	☐	☐	☐
7. Should the furniture be spaced wide enough for wheelchairs?	☐	☐	☐	☐
8. Should there be a quiet lounge with no television?	☐	☐	☐	☐ 20

Part VI: Recreational and Dining Areas

1. Should the dining room provide a choice of small and large tables to sit at?	☐	☐	☐	☐
2. Should the aisle space between tables in the dining room be wide enough for a wheelchair?	☐	☐	☐	☐
3. Should there be a library from which books can be borrowed?	☐	☐	☐	☐
4. Should there be a music or listening room?	☐	☐	☐	☐

Should the following recreational
or special activity materials be available?

5. Pool or billiard table?	☐	☐	☐	☐ 25
6. Ping-pong table?	☐	☐	☐	☐
7. Piano or organ?	☐	☐	☐	☐

	Not Important	Desirable	Very Important	Essential
	1	2	3	4
8. One or more television sets?	☐	☐	☐	☐
9. One or more phonographs?	☐	☐	☐	☐
10. One or more radios?	☐	☐	☐	☐
11. One or more sewing machines?	☐	☐	☐	☐ 31

Part VII: General Facilities

	Not Important	Desirable	Very Important	Essential
1. Should a map showing community resource be available in a convenient location?	☐	☐	☐	☐ 32
2. Should there be a bulletin board in a public location?	☐	☐	☐	☐
3. Should there be a posted list of the staff?	☐	☐	☐	☐
3a. If so, should it include pictures?	☐	☐	☐	☐ 35
4. Should there be a posted list of residents?	☐	☐	☐	☐
4a. If so, should it include pictures?	☐	☐	☐	☐
5. Should there be a sound system or public address system?	☐	☐	☐	☐
6. Should there be an air-conditioning system?	☐	☐	☐	☐
7. Should there be a chapel or meditation room?	☐	☐	☐	☐ 40
8. Should there be a gift shop or store?	☐	☐	☐	☐
9. Should residents and their visitors have access to a kitchen area?	☐	☐	☐	☐
10. Should there be a snack bar?	☐	☐	☐	☐
11. Should there be vending machines for candy or soft drinks for residents' use?	☐	☐	☐	☐
12. Should there be a laundry area for residents' use?	☐	☐	☐	☐ 45

Part VIII: Bathroom and Toilet Areas

	Not Important	Desirable	Very Important	Essential
	1	2	3	4
1. Should the bathroom doors open out?	☐	☐	☐	☐ 1
2. Should the threshold to the bathroom be level so that walkers or wheelchairs can enter easily?	☐	☐	☐	☐
3. Should there be handrails or safety bars in the bathroom?	☐	☐	☐	☐
4. Should there be lift bars next to the toilet?	☐	☐	☐	☐
5. Should the towel racks and dispensers be accessible to residents in wheelchairs?	☐	☐	☐	☐ 5
6. Should there be a mirror in every bathroom?	☐	☐	☐	☐
7. Should there be nonslip surfaces in all areas that may get wet?	☐	☐	☐	☐
8. Should there be a call button in every bathroom?	☐	☐	☐	☐
9. Should there be turning radius for a wheelchair in the bathroom (a 5-foot circle)?	☐	☐	☐	☐
10. Should there be a flexible shower (i.e., the shower head is mounted on the end of a long flexible hose to make bathing easier)?	☐	☐	☐	☐ 10
11. Should a seat be included in the shower?	☐	☐	☐	☐
12. Should a wheelchair-entered shower be available in some rooms or apartments?	☐	☐	☐	☐
13. Should each resident have access to both a bathtub and a shower?	☐	☐	☐	☐ 13

Part IX: Individual Rooms or Apartments

	Not Important	Desirable	Very Important	Essential
1. Should residents be able to hang pictures on the walls of their room or apartment?	☐	☐	☐	☐ 14
2. Should there be wall lights (or table lamps) that give adequate light for reading?	☐	☐	☐	☐
3. Should there be a mirror in every room or apartment?	☐	☐	☐	☐

	Not Important	Desirable	Very Important	Essential
	1	2	3	4
4. Should there be at least one window-sill that is wide enough to hold flowers?..... ☐	☐	☐	☐	
5. Should the floors be a light color? .... ☐	☐	☐	☐	
6. Should the walls be a light color? .... ☐	☐	☐	☐	
7. Should there be individual heating controls in all rooms or apartments? .... ☐	☐	☐	☐ 20	
8. Should there be individual air-conditioning controls in all rooms or apartments? .... ☐	☐	☐	☐	
9. Should residents be able to have a telephone in their rooms? .... ☐	☐	☐	☐	
10. Should there be enough space for wheelchair use in the rooms or apartments?................. ☐	☐	☐	☐	
11. Should there be handrails in the rooms?..... ☐	☐	☐	☐	
12. Should there be smoke detection devices in the rooms?... ☐	☐	☐	☐	
13. Should there be a call button in every room? ☐	☐	☐	☐ 26	

Part X: Staff and Office Areas

	Not Important	Desirable	Very Important	Essential
1. Should there be private offices for administrative staff?............................... ☐	☐	☐	☐ 27	
2. Should there be office space for secretarial and clerical staff? .... ☐	☐	☐	☐	
3. Should there be offices for social service and counseling staff? .... ☐	☐	☐	☐	
4. Should there be additional office space for other staff (e.g., activity director, volunteers, or part-time staff)? .... ☐	☐	☐	☐ 30	
5. Should the offices be free of distractions?... ☐	☐	☐	☐	
6. Should there be a separate room for handling mail, copying, and printing?....................... ☐	☐	☐	☐	
7. Should there be a conference room?........... ☐	☐	☐	☐	
8. Should there be a staff lounge?.................. ☐	☐	☐	☐	
8a. If so, should it have tables? .... ☐	☐	☐	☐	
8b. Should it have comfortable chairs? .... ☐	☐	☐	☐	
8c. Should the lounge be large enough to accommodate at least half the staff at one time? .... ☐	☐	☐	☐ 37	

POLICY AND PROGRAM INFORMATION FORM—
FORM I

In the next few years, new types of housing will be designed for older adults. We want to know what you think is most important in an *ideal* group living setting for older adults. Please answer the questions to describe the *best possible* living environment.

Many older adults find that they can no longer live alone in their own home. This may happen because they are in poor health, because their husband or wife has died, because it has become too expensive to keep up a house, or because of some combination of these factors. In such a situation, one alternative is to move to a group living setting in which there are rooms or apartments and in which meals are provided.

If the above statement described your situation, what would the *best possible* place for you be like? We would like you to tell us whether each policy or program feature would be part of an *ideal* setting for you.

Some questions will ask you to decide whether a particular policy or program feature should "definitely not," "preferably not," "preferably yes," or "definitely yes" be part of an ideal setting for you.

Other questions will ask whether a program feature is "not important," "desirable," "very important," or "essential" in an ideal setting. Place an "X" in the box for the answer that best describes your *ideal* setting. Please be sure to answer every question. Thank you for your help.

Your name (optional) _____ Date _____

Your age _____   Male ☐   Female ☐

Where do you live now? _____

How long have you lived there? _____

Part I: Expectations About Abilities

	Definitely Not	Preferably Not	Preferably Yes	Definitely Yes
	1	2	3	4

Should the following resident behaviors be tolerated?

1. Being unable to make one's own bed .... ☐ ☐ ☐ ☐ 1
2. Being unable to walk without assistance ..... ☐ ☐ ☐ ☐
3. Being unable to clean one's own room .... ☐ ☐ ☐ ☐
4. Being unable to feed oneself .... ☐ ☐ ☐ ☐
5. Being unable to bathe oneself .... ☐ ☐ ☐ ☐ 5
6. Being unable to dress oneself .... ☐ ☐ ☐ ☐
7. Being incontinent (of urine or feces) .... ☐ ☐ ☐ ☐
8. Being confused or disoriented .... ☐ ☐ ☐ ☐
9. Being depressed, crying frequently .... ☐ ☐ ☐ ☐
10. Refusing to participate in activities .... ☐ ☐ ☐ ☐ 10
11. Refusing to take prescribed medicine .... ☐ ☐ ☐ ☐
12. Taking medicine other than that which is prescribed .... ☐ ☐ ☐ ☐

Part II: Rules and Behaviors

Should the following be allowed?

1. Drinking liquor in one's own room .... ☐ ☐ ☐ ☐
2. Having one's own furniture in the room .... ☐ ☐ ☐ ☐
3. Moving furniture around the room .... ☐ ☐ ☐ ☐
4. Keeping a fish or bird in the room .... ☐ ☐ ☐ ☐ 16
5. Keeping a hot plate or coffee maker in the room .... ☐ ☐ ☐ ☐ 17
6. Doing some laundry in the bathroom .... ☐ ☐ ☐ ☐
7. Drinking a glass of wine or beer at meals .... ☐ ☐ ☐ ☐
8. Skipping breakfast to sleep late .... ☐ ☐ ☐ ☐ 20

Part III: Services and Procedures

	Definitely Not	Preferably Not	Preferably Yes	Definitely Yes
	1	2	3	4
1. If meals are provided, should there be at least an hour's range during which residents can choose to eat				
1a. Breakfast?	☐	☐	☐	☐
1b. Lunch?	☐	☐	☐	☐
1c. Dinner?	☐	☐	☐	☐
2. Should residents be able to sit wherever they want at meals?	☐	☐	☐	☐
3. Should residents be able to get up in the morning whenever they wish?	☐	☐	☐	☐ 25
4. Should residents be able to schedule baths or showers whenever they wish?	☐	☐	☐	☐
5. Should residents be able to go to bed at night whenever they wish?	☐	☐	☐	☐
6. Should residents be able to stay out in the evening as late as they wish?	☐	☐	☐	☐
7. Should all public areas of the building be open to residents at all times?	☐	☐	☐	☐
8. Should visiting hours allow for at least 11 hours of visiting a day?	☐	☐	☐	☐
9. Should a staff member take attendance or count residents at mealtimes?	☐	☐	☐	☐ 31
10. Should the staff check each day to make sure that none of the residents are missing?	☐	☐	☐	☐ 32
11. Should background music be played in the building?	☐	☐	☐	☐

Part IV: Rules About Problem Behaviors

As a general rule, should residents who persist in the following behaviors be allowed to remain in the facility?

1. Intentionally taking too much medicine	☐	☐	☐	☐
2. Being drunk	☐	☐	☐	☐ 35

	Definitely Not	Preferably Not	Preferably Yes	Definitely Yes
	1	2	3	4
3. Wandering around the building or grounds at night	☐	☐	☐	☐
4. Leaving the building during the evening without letting anyone know	☐	☐	☐	☐
5. Refusing to bathe or clean oneself regularly	☐	☐	☐	☐
6. Creating a disturbance; being noisy or boisterous	☐	☐	☐	☐
7. Stealing other residents' belongings	☐	☐	☐	☐ 40
8. Damaging or destroying property (e.g., tearing books or magazines)	☐	☐	☐	☐
9. Verbally threatening another resident	☐	☐	☐	☐
10. Physically attacking another resident	☐	☐	☐	☐
11. Physically attacking a staff member	☐	☐	☐	☐
12. Attempting suicide	☐	☐	☐	☐
13. Indecently exposing themselves	☐	☐	☐	☐ 46

Part V: Resident Participation

1. Should any of the residents be hired and paid for jobs in the building?	☐	☐	☐	☐ 47
2. Should residents be able to perform chores or duties (unpaid) in the building if they wish?	☐	☐	☐	☐
2a. Should at least 10% of the residents be involved in chores around the facility?	☐	☐	☐	☐
3. Should there be a residents' council (i.e., residents who are elected to represent other residents at regular meetings)?	☐	☐	☐	☐ 50
3a. If so, should the residents' council meet at least twice a month?	☐	☐	☐	☐
3b. Should there be at least one representative on the residents' council for every 25 residents?	☐	☐	☐	☐
4. Should there be regular "house meetings" for residents (a general meeting open to all residents)?	☐	☐	☐	☐
4a. If so, should the house meetings occur at least once a month?	☐	☐	☐	☐

	Definitely Not	Preferably Not	Preferably Yes	Definitely Yes
	1	2	3	4
5. Should there be one or more committees that include residents as members?	☐	☐	☐	☐ 55
5a. Should committees meet at least once a month?	☐	☐	☐	☐
5b. Should committees include at least 10% of the residents?	☐	☐	☐	☐
6. Should there be a newsletter primarily written by residents?	☐	☐	☐	☐
7. Should there be a bulletin board that is used by residents?	☐	☐	☐	☐ 59

Part VI: Decision Making

Should residents be *largely responsible* for

1. Planning entertainment such as movies or parties?	☐	☐	☐	☐ 1
2. Planning educational activities such as courses and lectures?	☐	☐	☐	☐
3. Planning welcoming or orientation activities?	☐	☐	☐	☐
4. Deciding what kinds of new activities or programs will occur?	☐	☐	☐	☐
5. Making rules about attendance at activities?	☐	☐	☐	☐ 5

Should residents have *at least some responsibility* for

6. Planning daily or weekly menus?	☐	☐	☐	☐
7. Setting mealtimes?	☐	☐	☐	☐
8. Setting visitors' hours?	☐	☐	☐	☐
9. Deciding on the decor of public areas (e.g., pictures in halls, plants, etc.)?	☐	☐	☐	☐
10. Dealing with safety hazards?	☐	☐	☐	☐ 10
11. Dealing with residents' complaints?	☐	☐	☐	☐
12. Making rules about the use of alcohol?	☐	☐	☐	☐

	Definitely Not	Preferably Not	Preferably Yes	Definitely Yes
	1	2	3	4
13. Selecting new residents?	☐	☐	☐	☐
14. Moving a resident from one bed or room to another?	☐	☐	☐	☐
15. Deciding when a troublesome or sick resident should be asked to leave?	☐	☐	☐	☐
16. Changes in staff (hiring or firing)?	☐	☐	☐	☐ 16

Part VII: Types of Rooms and Privacy

	1	2	3	4
1. Should every resident have the option of a private room?	☐	☐	☐	☐ 17
2. Should every resident have the option of a private bathroom?	☐	☐	☐	☐
3. Consider a situation in which some residents must share rooms:				
3a. Should there be a limit of two persons who share a bedroom or apartment?	☐	☐	☐	☐
3b. Should there be a limit of two persons who share a bathroom?	☐	☐	☐	☐ 20
4. Should residents have their own private mailboxes?	☐	☐	☐	☐
5. Should each resident be allowed to have a separate dresser?	☐	☐	☐	☐
6. Should there be locks on all bathroom doors?	☐	☐	☐	☐
7. Should residents be able to close the door to their room or apartment?	☐	☐	☐	☐
8. Should residents be able to lock the door to their room or apartment?	☐	☐	☐	☐ 25
9. Should there be private staff offices that can be used for interviewing residents?	☐	☐	☐	☐

Part VIII: Policies and General Information

	1	2	3	4
1. Should there be an orientation handbook for residents?	☐	☐	☐	☐
2. Should there be an orientation handbook for staff?	☐	☐	☐	☐

	Definitely Not	Preferably Not	Preferably Yes	Definitely Yes
	1	2	3	4
3. Should there be an orientation program for new residents?	☐	☐	☐	☐
4. Should there be an orientation program for new staff?	☐	☐	☐	☐ 30
5. Should there be formal staff meetings?	☐	☐	☐	☐ 31
5a. If so, should the staff meetings be held at least once a week?	☐	☐	☐	☐
6. If there are volunteers, should they have an orientation program?	☐	☐	☐	☐
7. Should there be a newsletter?	☐	☐	☐	☐
7a. If so, should the newsletter be printed at least once a month?	☐	☐	☐	☐ 35
8. Should rules and regulations be posted on the bulletin board or in another convenient public location?	☐	☐	☐	☐

Part IX: Health Services

Should the following health services be provided?

1. Regularly scheduled doctor's hours	☐	☐	☐	☐
2. Doctor on call	☐	☐	☐	☐
3. Regularly scheduled nurse's hours	☐	☐	☐	☐
4. Assistance in using prescribed medications	☐	☐	☐	☐ 40
5. On-site medical clinic	☐	☐	☐	☐
6. Physical therapy	☐	☐	☐	☐
7. Occupational therapy	☐	☐	☐	☐
8. Psychotherapy or personal counseling	☐	☐	☐	☐ 44

Part X: Assistance in Daily Living

Should the following services to aid daily living be provided?

1. Assistance with housekeeping or cleaning	☐	☐	☐	☐ 45
2. Assistance with personal care or grooming	☐	☐	☐	☐
3. Religious advice or counseling	☐	☐	☐	☐
4. Legal advice or counseling	☐	☐	☐	☐

	Definitely Not	Preferably Not	Preferably Yes	Definitely Yes
	1	2	3	4
5. Assistance with banking or other financial matters	☐	☐	☐	☐ 50
6. Barber or beauty service	☐	☐	☐	☐
7. Assistance with laundry or linen service	☐	☐	☐	☐
8. Assistance with shopping	☐	☐	☐	☐
9. Transportation (e.g., minibus or pickup car)	☐	☐	☐	☐
10. Handling spending money for residents	☐	☐	☐	☐
11. Serving breakfast every day	☐	☐	☐	☐ 55
12. Serving lunch every day	☐	☐	☐	☐
13. Serving dinner every day	☐	☐	☐	☐
14. Serving snacks in the afternoon or evening.	☐	☐	☐	☐ 58

Part XI: Facility Activities

Should the following social and recreational activities be provided *at least twice a month?*

	Definitely Not	Preferably Not	Preferably Yes	Definitely Yes
1. Exercises or other physical fitness activity	☐	☐	☐	☐ 1
2. Outside entertainment (e.g., pianist or singer)	☐	☐	☐	☐
3. Discussion groups	☐	☐	☐	☐
4. Reality orientation group	☐	☐	☐	☐
5. Self-help or mutual support group	☐	☐	☐	☐ 5
6. Films or movies	☐	☐	☐	☐
7. Clubs, social groups, or drama or singing groups	☐	☐	☐	☐
8. Classes or lectures	☐	☐	☐	☐
9. Bingo, cards, or other games	☐	☐	☐	☐
10. Parties	☐	☐	☐	☐ 10
11. Religious services	☐	☐	☐	☐
12. Social hour (e.g., coffee or cocktail hour)	☐	☐	☐	☐
13. Arts and crafts	☐	☐	☐	☐ 13

SHELTERED CARE ENVIRONMENT SCALE
FORM I

Name (optional)_____ Age_____

Name of facility_____

    Male ☐   Female ☐

How long have you lived or worked here? _____ _____ _____

                                  Years   Months   Days

If you are a staff member, check the following box ☐
and indicate your staff position _____

Today's date _____

    There are 63 questions here. They ask what you think an *ideal* residential setting would be like. You are to decide which statements would be true of an ideal residential setting and which would be false.

    Circle yes if you think the statement is true or mostly true of an *ideal* residential setting.

    Circle no if you think the statement is false or mostly false of an *ideal* residential setting.

    Please be sure to answer every question. Thank you for your cooperation.

1. Will residents get a lot of individual attention? ....Yes No

2. Will residents ever start arguments?...Yes No

3. Will residents usually depend on the staff to set up
   activities for them?...Yes No

4. Will residents be careful about what they say to each other?........Yes No

5. Will residents always know when the staff will be around?..........Yes No

6. Will the staff be strict about rules and regulations? ....Yes No

7. Will the furniture be comfortable and homey? ....Yes No

8. Will staff members spend a lot of time with residents?................Yes No

9. Will it be unusual for residents to openly express their anger?....Yes No

10. Will residents usually wait for staff to suggest an idea
    or activity? ....Yes No

11. Will personal problems be openly talked about? ....Yes No

12. Will activities for residents be carefully planned? ....Yes No

13. Will new and different ideas often be tried out?...........................Yes No

14. Will it ever be cold and drafty?...Yes No

15. Will staff members sometimes talk down to residents?................Yes No

16. Will residents sometimes criticize or make fun of the place?.......Yes No

17. Will residents be taught how to deal with practical problems?....Yes No

18. Will residents tend to hide their feelings from one another? ....Yes No

19. Will some residents look messy? ....Yes No

20. If two residents fight with each other, will they get in trouble?...Yes No

21. Will residents have privacy whenever they want? ....Yes No

22. Will there be a lot of social activities?...Yes No

23. Will residents usually keep their disagreements to themselves? ...Yes No

24. Will many new skills be taught? ....Yes No

25. Will residents talk a lot about their fears?......................................Yes No

26. Will things always seem to be changing?.......................................Yes No

27. Will staff allow the residents to break minor rules?......................Yes No

28. Will the place seem crowded?..Yes No

29. Will a lot of the residents just seem to be passing time? ....Yes No

30. Will it be unusual for residents to complain about each other? ...Yes   No

31. Will residents be learning to do more things on their own? ....Yes   No

32. Will it be hard to tell how the residents are feeling?....................Yes   No

33. Will residents know what will happen to them if they
    break a rule? ....Yes   No

34. Will suggestions made by the residents be acted on? ....Yes   No

35. Will it sometimes be very noisy? ....Yes   No

36. Will requests made by residents usually be taken care of
    right away?..Yes   No

37. Will it always be peaceful and quiet? ....Yes   No

38. Will the residents be strongly encouraged to make their own
    decisions? ....Yes   No

39. Will residents talk a lot about their past dreams and
    ambitions?...Yes   No

40. Will there be a lot of confusion at times?......................................Yes   No

41. Will residents have any say in making the rules? ....Yes   No

42. Will it ever smell bad?..Yes   No

43. Will staff members sometimes criticize residents over
    minor things? ....Yes   No

44. Will residents often get impatient with each other?.....................Yes   No

45. Will residents sometimes take charge of activities? ....Yes   No

46. Will residents ever talk about illness and death?...........................Yes   No

47. Will the place be very well organized? ....Yes   No

48. Will the rules and regulations be rather strictly enforced?...........Yes   No

49. Will it ever be hot and stuffy? ....Yes   No

50. Will residents tend to keep to themselves?....................................Yes   No

51. Will residents complain a lot? ....Yes   No

52. Will residents care more about the past than the future?.............Yes   No

53. Will residents talk about their money problems? ....Yes   No

54. Will things sometimes be unclear? ....Yes   No

55. Will a resident ever be asked to leave if he or she breaks a rule? ......Yes   No

56. Will the lighting be very good? ....Yes   No

57. Will the discussions be very interesting? ....Yes   No

58. Will residents criticize each other a lot?........................Yes   No

59. Will some of the residents' activities be really challenging?.........Yes   No

60. Will residents keep their personal problems to themselves? ....Yes   No

61. Will people always be changing their minds?...............................Yes   No

62. Will residents be able to change things if they really try? ....Yes   No

63. Will the colors and decorations make the place warm
    and cheerful?..Yes   No

FORM I SCORING DIRECTIONS

Form I of the PAF and POLIF can be scored dichotomously or on a 4-point scale. Using dichotomous scoring, score responses of not important and desirable (or of definitely not and preferably not) as 0 points; score responses of very important and essential (or of preferably yes and definitely yes) as 1 point. Note that the scoring of all items on Expectations for Functioning and one item on Policy Choice is reversed (see POLIF Form I Scoring Key). For these items, definitely not and preferably not are scored 1.

Add up the item scores to get the subscale total; divide the total score by the number of items on the subscale and multiply by 100 to compute the percentage score. The percentage scores can be compared with the normative scores shown in Chapters 4 and 5.

Using 4-point scoring, give more weight to the more positive responses. That is, score a response of definitely not or not important as 0 points, preferably not or desirable as 1 point, preferably yes or very important as 2 points, and definitely yes or essential as 3 points. Again, the exception is the scoring of all items on Expectations for Functioning and one item on Policy Choice, which is reversed.

As in the dichotomous scoring, add the item scores to get the subscale total. To compute the percentage score, divide the subscale score by the total number of possible points on the subscale—that is, three times the number of items on the subscale and multiply by 100. The percentage scores can be compared with the normative scores shown in Tables D.1 through D.3.

PAF Form I Scoring Key

1. *Community Accessibility*

   Part I: Items 1a, 1b, 1c, 1d, 1e, 1f, 1g, 1h, 1i, 1j, 1k, 1l, 2, 3, 3a, 4

2. *Physical Amenities*

   Part II: Items 1, 4c, 6b, 6c, 6d, 6e, 8
   Part IV: Items 4, 5, 5b, 6, 6a, 6d
   Part V: Item 6
   Part VII: Items 6, 7, 8, 9, 11, 12
   Part VIII: Items 6, 13
   Part IX: Items 1, 2, 3, 4, 5, 6, 7, 8

3. *Social-Recreational Aids*

   Part II: Items 4, 4d, 5, 6a, 6f, 6g, 7, 11
   Part III: Items 11, 12
   Part V: Items 1, 2, 3, 4, 5, 8
   Part VI: Items 1, 3, 4, 5, 6, 7, 8, 9, 10, 11
   Part VII: Item 10
   Part IX: Item 9

4. *Prosthetic Aids*

   Part II: Item 9
   Part III: Items 1, 5, 6, 7
   Part IV: Items 1, 3, 5a, 6b, 6c, 8
   Part V: Item 7
   Part VI: Item 2
   Part VIII: Items 1, 2, 3, 4, 5, 9, 10, 11, 12
   Part IX: Items 10, 11

5. *Orientational Aids*

   Part III: Items 4, 9, 14
   Part IV: Items 11, 12, 13
   Part VII: Items 1, 2, 3, 3a, 4, 4a, 5

6. *Safety Features*

   Part II: Items 2, 3a, 3b, 4a, 4b
   Part III: Items 2, 3, 8, 10, 13
   Part IV: Items 2, 7, 9, 10
   Part VIII: Items 7, 8
   Part IX: Items 12, 13

7. *Staff Facilities*

   Part II: Item 10
   Part X: Items 2, 3, 4, 5, 6, 7, 8, 8a, 8b, 8c

POLIF Form I Scoring Key

1. *Expectations for Functioning* (reverse scoring on all items)

   Part I: Items 1, 2, 3, 4, 5, 6, 7, 8, 9
   Part III: Items 9, 10

2. *Acceptance of Problem Behavior*

   Part I: Items 10, 11, 12
   Part IV: Items 1, 2, 3, 4, 5, 6, 7, 8, 9, 10, 11, 12, 13

3. *Policy Choice*

   Part II: Items 1, 2, 3, 4, 5, 6, 7, 8
   Part III: Items 1a, 1b, 1c, 2, 3, 4, 5, 6, 7, 8, 11 (reverse score item)

4. *Resident Control*

   Part V: Items 1, 2, 2a, 3, 3a, 3b, 4, 4a, 5, 5a, 5b, 6, 7
   Part VI: Items 1, 2, 3, 4, 5, 6, 7, 8, 9, 10, 11, 12, 13, 14, 15, 16

5. *Policy Clarity*

   Part VIII: Items 1, 2, 3, 4, 5, 5a, 6, 7, 7a, 8

6. *Provision for Privacy*

   Part VII: Items 1, 2, 3a, 3b, 4, 5, 6, 7, 8, 9

7. *Availability of Health Services*

   Part IX: Items 1, 2, 3, 4, 5, 6, 7, 8

8. *Availability of Daily Living Assistance*

   Part X: Items 1, 2, 3, 4, 5, 6, 7, 8, 9, 10, 11, 12, 13, 14

9. *Availability of Social-Recreational Activities*

   Part XI: Items 1, 2, 3, 4, 5, 6, 7, 8, 9, 10, 11, 12, 13

Form I Norms on 4-Point Scales

TABLE D.1 PAF and POLIF Form I Subscale Means and Standard Deviations for the Total Sample and Three Subsamples of Residents (4-Point Scale)

Subscale	Total Sample of Residents (n = 422)		Nursing Home Residents (n = 40)		Residential Care Residents (n = 153)		Apartment Residents (n = 229)	
	Mean	SD	Mean	SD	Mean	SD	Mean	SD
PAF Form I								
Community Accessibility	53	20	34	21	56	21	53	18
Physical Amenities	50	15	49	13	53	17	49	14
Social-Recreational Aids	43	15	43	13	45	17	42	13
Prosthetic Aids	56	16	68	13	59	17	52	15
Orientational Aids	50	17	45	13	52	19	50	16
Safety Features	64	17	63	14	64	20	65	15
Staff Facilities	46	21	50	16	49	23	43	19
POLIF Form I								
Expectations for Functioning	63	24	19	19	61	18	1	19
Acceptance of Problem Behavior	15	16	28	22	16	17	13	12
Policy Choice	64	16	50	12	58	14	71	14
Resident Control	54	17	43	16	61	16	51	15
Policy Clarity	53	22	49	19	59	23	50	21
Provision for Privacy	66	23	39	16	58	22	76	17
Health Services Availability	45	27	55	20	61	25	34	23
Daily Living Assistance Availability	38	20	58	14	43	20	32	18
Social-Recreational Activities Availability	41	20	48	18	44	24	38	17

TABLE D.2 PAF and POLIF Form I Subscale Means and Standard
Deviations for the Total Sample and Three Subsamples of Staff
(4-Point Scale)

Subscale	Total Sample of Staff (n = 98)		Nursing Home Staff (n = 33)		Residential Care Staff (n = 34)		Apartment Staff (n = 31)	
	Mean	SD	Mean	SD	Mean	SD	Mean	SD
PAF Form I								
Community Accessibility	50	17	47	22	50	17	53	9
Physical Amenities	58	14	62	13	58	13	53	15
Social-Recreational Aids	53	16	56	16	53	16	50	15
Prosthetic Aids	61	15	69	12	59	14	56	17
Orientational Aids	53	16	56	16	52	16	52	15
Safety Features	69	14	69	13	70	16	67	14
Staff Facilities	66	21	73	19	63	22	61	22
POLIF Form I								
Expectations for Functioning	49	29	17	20	58	15	74	16
Acceptance of Problem Behavior	26	19	29	15	16	12	32	25
Policy Choice	65	17	56	19	65	14	74	13
Resident Control	52	15	51	18	50	14	54	13
Policy Clarity	62	19	65	17	58	20	61	20
Provision for Privacy	66	23	47	17	70	22	81	13
Health Services Availability	48	27	69	12	44	25	30	24
Daily Living Assistance Availability	55	25	73	18	58	17	32	21
Social-Recreational Activities Availability	63	22	75	20	60	21	54	21

TABLE D.3 PAF and POLIF Form I Subscale Means and Standard Deviations for Potential Residents and Experts (4-Point Scale)

Subscale	Potential Nursing Home Residents (n = 30)		Potential Apartment Residents (n = 205)		Experts (n = 44)	
	Mean	SD	Mean	SD	Mean	SD
PAF Form I						
Community Accessibility	52	17	52	17	57	12
Physical Amenities	48	13	52	16	65	12
Social-Recreational Aids	43	14	44	15	56	13
Prosthetic Aids	66	19	61	16	72	13
Orientational Aids	47	15	51	18	61	17
Safety Features	67	14	67	17	72	12
Staff Facilities	54	21	45	23	54	20
POLIF Form I						
Expectations for Functioning	45	36	60	28	47	23
Acceptance of Problem Behavior	9	16	10	14	38	26
Policy Choice	69	17	78	18	96	7
Resident Control	60	19	73	22	90	11
Policy Clarity	57	27	53	31	75	22
Provision for Privacy	63	22	69	26	89	14
Health Services Availability	50	36	45	36	57	29
Daily Living Assistance Availability	35	32	29	26	56	25
Social-Recreational Activities Availability	28	30	31	31	59	28

Appendix E: Service Utilization Dimensions— Scoring Key and Norms

The questions about numbers of residents using services or participating in activities, which are contained in Section IV of the Policy and Program Information Form (POLIF), constitute three service utilization dimensions. They are considered an optional part of the POLIF and an adjunct to the Resident and Staff Information Form (RESIF).

Utilization of Health Services measures the proportion of residents who use each of the health services that the facility offers. Daily Living Assistance Utilization provides information on the proportion of residents who use such facility services as assistance with housekeeping, personal care, shopping, and transportation. It taps a somewhat different aspect of resident functioning than the Functional Abilities subscale of the RESIF because residents who need assistance may not use it and the assistance itself may not be provided by the facility. Finally, Social-Recreational Activities Utilization assesses resident participation in the activities offered in the facility such as parties, discussion groups, and classes. These subscales provide descriptive information about the resident population and about program use and can be used to measure resident outcomes (e.g., see Moos & Lemke, 1994).

For directions on obtaining this information, see Chapter 5. This appendix contains information on the psychometric characteristics of these subscales, directions for hand scoring, and tables of means and standard deviations for these subscales in the normative samples of community and veterans facilities.

TABLE E.1 Means and Standard Deviations of the Service Utilization Dimensions for the Total Community Sample and the Three Subsamples

Subscale	Total Sample (n = 262 Facilities)		Nursing Homes (n = 135 Facilities)		Residential Care (n = 60 Facilities)		Apartments (n = 67 Facilities)	
	Mean	SD	Mean	SD	Mean	SD	Mean	SD
Utilization of Health Services	41	23	50	11	43	29	9	7
Utilization of Daily Living Assistance	58	22	68	10	64	19	31	22
Utilization of Social-Recreational Activities	42	22	43	17	55	25	29	19

TABLE E.2 Means and Standard Deviations of the Service Utilization Dimensions for the Total Veterans Sample and the Two Subsamples

Subscale	Total Sample (n = 81 Facilities)		Nursing Care Units (n = 57 Facilities)		Domiciliaries (n = 24 Facilities)	
	Mean	SD	Mean	SD	Mean	SD
Utilization of Health Services	41	13	47	92	6	8
Utilization of Daily Living Assistance	59	13	61	9	54	19
Utilization of Social-Recreational Activities	40	16	43	16	33	15

PSYCHOMETRIC CHARACTERISTICS

Internal consistencies in a subset of more than 140 community facilities range from moderate ($r = .67$ for Health Services Utilization) to high (r above .80 for the remaining two dimensions). All three subscales show high test-retest stability (r above .75 for 9- to 12-month test-retest reliability in a sample of 12 facilities).

Although the dimensions are conceptually distinct, there are moderate empirical relationships among them (r ranges from .33 to .49 among the three subscales in the community sample).

NORMATIVE DATA

The means and standard deviations of the three utilization dimensions are given in Table E.1 for the total community sample and three subsamples and in Table E.2 for the total veterans sample and two subsamples.

HAND-SCORING WORKSHEETS

Before scoring the utilization dimensions, be sure that all relevant information has been converted to percentage of total residents. Transfer the information from the POLIF (section and item number are indicated for each question). Circle "n.a." if the service is not available.

1. Utilization of Health Services

Section IV, Part I   Percentage

Approximately what percentage of the residents
use the following services at least once in a typical week?

1. Regularly scheduled doctor's hours .... n.a. _____

2. Doctor on call .... n.a. _____

3. Regularly scheduled nurse's hours .... n.a. _____

4. Assistance in using prescribed medications .... n.a. _____

5. On-site medical clinic... n.a._____

6. Physical therapy .... n.a._____

7. Occupational therapy.. n.a. _____

8. Psychotherapy or personal counseling .... n.a. _____

SCORING: Add the numbers in the percentage column and enter the sum as the total score. To obtain the total points possible, subtract the total number of n.a.s from 8. To compute the percentage score, divide the total score by the total points possible.

_____ ÷ _____ = _____
(total score)   (total points possible)   (percentage score)

2. *Utilization of Daily Living Assistance*

Section IV, Part I   Percentage

Approximately what percentage of the
residents use the following services?

  9. Religious advice or counseling .... n.a. _____

10. Legal advice or counseling .... n.a. _____

11. Assistance with banking or other financial matters .... n.a. _____

12. Assistance with housekeeping or cleaning .... n.a. _____

14. Assistance with personal care or grooming .... n.a. _____

15. Barber or beauty service .... n.a. _____

16. Assistance with laundry or linen service .... n.a. _____

17. Assistance with shopping .... n.a. _____

18. Providing transportation (e.g., minibus or pickup car) .... n.a. _____

19. Handling spending money for residents .... n.a. _____

Section IV, Part II (p. 000)

1b. Breakfast .... n.a. _____

2b. Lunch .... n.a. _____

4a. Afternoon or evening snacks .... n.a. _____

Section IV, Part I (POLIF)

13. Assistance with preparing meals OR

Section IV, Part II

3b. Dinner .... n.a. _____

**SCORING: Add the numbers in the percentage column and enter the sum as the
total score. To obtain the total points possible, subtract the total number of n.a.s
from 14. To compute the percentage score, divide the total score by the total
points possible.**

    _____ ÷ _____ = _____

    (total score)   (total points possible)   (percentage score)

3. Utilization of Social-Recreational Activities

Section IV, Part III   Percentage

About what percentage of the residents participate
in the following activities? If the activity is offered
only a few times a year or less, circle n.a. and
do not give a percentage for participation.

1. Exercise or other physical fitness activity.................................... n.a. _____

2. Outside entertainment (e.g., pianist or singer).......................... n.a. _____

3. Discussion groups .... n.a. _____

4. Reality orientation group... n.a. _____

5. Self-help or mutual support group... n.a. _____

6. Films or movies.. n.a. _____

7. Club, social group, or drama or singing groups .... n.a. _____

8. Classes or lectures .... n.a. _____

9. Bingo, cards, or other games.. n.a. _____

10. Parties .... n.a. _____

11. Religious services .... n.a. _____

12. Social hour (e.g., coffee or cocktail hour) .... n.a. _____

13. Arts and crafts... n.a. _____

**SCORING: Add the numbers in the percentage column and enter the sum as the
total score. To obtain the total points possible, subtract the total number of n.a.s
from 13. To compute the percentage score, divide the total score by the total
points possible.**

_____ ÷ _____ = _____
(total score)   (total points possible)   (percentage score)

REFERENCES

Benjamin, L. C., & Spector, J. (1990). Environments for the dementing. *International Journal of Geriatric Psychiatry, 5,* 15-24.

Benjamin, L. C., & Spector, J. (1992). Geriatric care on a ward without nurses. *International Journal of Geriatric Psychiatry, 7,* 743-750.

Berkowitz, M. W., Waxman, R., & Yaffe, L. (1988). The effects of a resident self-help model on control, social involvement and self-esteem among the elderly. *The Gerontologist, 28,* 620-624.

Billingsley, J. D., & Batterson, C. T. (1986). Evaluating long-term care facilities: A field application of the MEAP. *Journal of Long-Term Care Administration, 14,* 16-19.

Blake, R. (1985-1986). Normalization and boarding homes: An examination of paradoxes. *Social Work in Health Care, 11,* 75-86.

Blake, R. (1987). The social environment of boarding homes. *Adult Foster Care Journal, 1,* 42-55.

Braun, B. I. (1991). The effect of nursing home quality on patient outcome. *Journal of the American Geriatrics Society, 39,* 329-338.

Braun, K. L., & Rose, C. L. (1989). Goals and characteristics of long-term care programs: An analytic model. *The Gerontologist, 29,* 51-58.

Brennan, P. L., & Moos, R. H. (1990). Physical design, social climate, and staff turnover in skilled nursing facilities. *Journal of Long-Term Care Administration, 18,* 22-27.

Brennan, P. L., Moos, R. H., & Lemke, S. (1988). Preferences of older adults and experts for physical and architectural features of group living facilities. *The Gerontologist, 28,* 84-90.

Brennan, P. L., Moos, R. H., & Lemke, S. (1989). Preferences of older adults and experts for policies and services in group living facilities. *Psychology and Aging, 4,* 48-56.

Byerts, T. O., & Heller, T. (1985). *Longitudinal research on congregate public housing* (Final Report). Chicago: University of Illinois, College of Architecture.

Campbell, V. A., & Bailey, C. J. (1984). Comparison of methods for classifying community residential settings for mentally retarded individuals. *American Journal of Mental Deficiency, 89,* 44-49.

327

Carp, F. M., & Carp, A. (1984). A complementary/congruence model of well-being or mental health for the community elderly. In I. Altman, M. P. Lawton, & J. F. Wohlwill (Eds.), *Elderly people and the environment* (pp. 279-336). New York: Plenum.

Chambers, L., Forchuk, C., Munroe-Blum, H., Woodcox, V., Moore, G., & Wigmore, D. (1988). The development of guidelines to promote a therapeutic environment in lodging homes. *Canada's Mental Health, 36,* 14-18.

Clark, H. M. (1989). A study of the relationships between personal characteristics, social environment and well-being in older nursing home residents (Doctoral dissertation, University of Maryland, College Park, 1988). *Dissertation Abstracts International, 50,* 1309B.

Colling, J. (1989). *Nursing home residents' well-being as related to their control of activities of daily living.* Portland: Oregon Health Sciences University, School of Nursing.

Conrad, K. J., Hanrahan, P., & Hughes, S. L. (1988). The use of profiles and models in evaluating program environments. In K. J. Conrad & C. Roberts-Gray (Eds.), *Evaluating program environments: New directions for program evaluation* (No. 40, pp. 25-43). San Francisco: Jossey-Bass.

Conrad, K. J., Hanrahan, P., & Hughes, S. L. (1990). Survey of adult day care in the United States: National and regional findings. *Research on Aging, 12,* 36-56.

Conrad, K. J., Hughes, S. L., Hanrahan, P., & Wang, S. (1993). Classification of adult day care: A cluster analysis of services and activities. *Journal of Gerontology: Social Sciences, 48,* S112-S122.

Conrad, K. J., & Miller, T. Q. (1987). Measuring and testing program philosophy. In L. Bickman (Ed.), *Using program theory in evaluation* (pp. 19-42). San Francisco: Jossey-Bass.

David, T. G., Moos, R. H., & Kahn, J. R. (1981). Community integration among elderly residents of sheltered care settings. *American Journal of Community Psychology, 9,* 513-526.

Deutschman, M. (1982). Environmental settings and environmental competence. *Gerontology and Geriatrics Education, 2,* 237-242.

Duncan, O. D. (1961). A socioeconomic index for all occupations. In A. J. Reiss (Ed.), *Occupations and social status* (pp. 109-138). New York: Free Press.

Earls, M., & Nelson, G. (1988). The relationship between long-term psychiatric clients' psychological well-being and their perceptions of housing and social support. *American Journal of Community Psychology, 16,* 279-293.

Fernandez-Ballesteros, R., Diaz, P., Izal, M., & Gonzalez, J. L. (1987). Evaluacion de una residencia de ancianos y valoracion de intervenciones ambientales. In R. Fernandez-Ballesteros (Ed.), *El ambiente analisis psicologico* (pp. 227-248). Madrid: Don Ramon de la Cruz.

Fernandez-Ballesteros, R., Izal, M., Diaz, P., Gonzalez, J. L., Vila, E., & Espinosa, M. J. (1986). Estudio ecopsicologico de una residencia de ancianos. In R. Fernandez-Ballesteros (Ed.), *Evaluacion de contextos* (pp. 59-103). Murcia, Spain: Servicio de Publicaciones, Universidad de Murcia.

Fernandez-Ballesteros, R., Izal, M., Montorio, I., Llorente, M. G., Hernandez, J. M., & Guerrero, M. A. (1991). Evaluation of residential programs for the elderly in Spain and the United States. *Evaluation Practice, 12,* 159-164.

Finney, J. W., & Moos, R. H. (1984). Environmental assessment and evaluation research: Examples from mental health and substance abuse programs. *Evaluation and Program Planning, 7,* 151-167.

Finney, J. W., & Moos, R. H. (1992). The long-term course of treated alcoholism: II. Predictors and correlates of 10-year functioning and mortality. *Journal of Studies on Alcohol, 53*, 142-153.

Garritson, S. H. (1987). Characteristics of restrictiveness. *Journal of Psychosocial Nursing, 25*, 10-19.

Hatcher, M., Gentry, R., Kunkel, M., & Smith, G. (1983). Environmental assessment and community intervention: An application of the social ecology model. *Psychosocial Rehabilitation Journal, 7*, 22-28.

Hodge, G. (1987). Assisted housing for Ontario's rural elderly: Shortfalls in product and location. *Canadian Journal on Aging, 6*, 141-154.

Izal, M. (1992). Residential facilities for older adults: Cross-cultural environmental assessment. *European Journal of Psychological Assessment, 8*, 118-134.

Johnson, P. D. (1981). Effects of increased personal and interpersonal control upon the well-being of institutionalized geriatrics (Doctoral dissertation, Arizona State University, Phoenix, 1981). *Dissertation Abstracts International, 42*, 748B.

Jones, J. P., & Batterson, C. T. (1982). *Quality of life survey*. Carmichael, CA: Eskaton Administrative Center.

Kodama, K. (1986). The development and the effectiveness of a rating scale for environmental features at residential facilities for the aged. *Journal of Architecture, Planning, and Environmental Engineering, 366*, 53-60.

Kodama, K. (1988a). The analysis of architectural complaints related to architectural conditions of the homes for the aged rated by the residents. *Journal of Architecture, Planning, and Environmental Engineering, 385*, 53-63.

Kodama, K. (1988b). How architectural conditions affect the morale and the environmental distress of the residents of old age homes. *Journal of Architecture, Planning, and Environmental Engineering, 390*, 77-85.

Kruzich, J. M., Clinton, J. F., & Kelber, S. T. (1992). Personal and environmental influences on nursing home satisfaction. *The Gerontologist, 32*, 342-350.

Lawton, M. P. (1982). Competence, environmental press, and the adaptation of older people. In M. P. Lawton, P. G. Windley, & T. O. Byerts (Eds.), *Aging and the environment: Theoretical approaches* (pp. 33-59). New York: Springer.

Lawton, M. P. (1989). Behavior-relevant ecological factors. In K. W. Schaie & C. Schoder (Eds.), *Social structure and aging: Psychological processes* (pp. 57-78). Hillsdale, NJ: Lawrence Erlbaum.

Lehman, A. F. (1988). A quality of life interview for the chronically mentally ill. *Evaluation and Program Planning, 11*, 51-62.

Lehman, A. F., Possidente, S., & Hawker, F. (1986). The quality of life of chronic patients in a state hospital and in community residences. *Hospital and Community Psychiatry, 37*, 901-907.

Lemke, S., & Moos, R. H. (1980). Assessing the institutional policies of sheltered care settings. *Journal of Gerontology, 35*, 96-107.

Lemke, S., & Moos, R. H. (1981). The suprapersonal environments of sheltered care settings. *Journal of Gerontology, 36*, 233-243.

Lemke, S., & Moos, R. H. (1984). Coping with an intra-institutional relocation: Behavioral change as a function of residents' personal resources. *Journal of Environmental Psychology, 4*, 137-151.

Lemke, S., & Moos, R. H. (1985). The evaluation process in housing for the elderly. In G. M. Gutman & M. K. Blackie (Eds.), *Innovations in housing and living environments for seniors* (pp. 227-254). Vancouver, Canada: Simon Fraser University, Gerontology Research Centre.

Lemke, S., & Moos, R. H. (1986). Quality of residential settings for elderly adults. *Journal of Gerontology, 41,* 268-276.

Lemke, S., & Moos, R. (1987). Measuring the social climate of congregate residences for older people: Sheltered Care Environment Scale. *Psychology and Aging, 2,* 20-29.

Lemke, S., & Moos, R. H. (1989a). Ownership and quality of care in residential facilities for the elderly. *The Gerontologist, 29,* 209-215.

Lemke, S., & Moos, R. H. (1989b). Personal and environmental determinants of activity involvement among elderly residents of congregate facilities. *Journal of Gerontology: Social Sciences, 44,* S139-S148.

Lemke, S., & Moos, R. H. (1990). Validity of the Sheltered Care Environment Scale: Conceptual and methodological issues. *Psychology and Aging, 5,* 569-571.

Linn, M. W., Gurel, L., Williford, W. O., Overall, J., Gurland, B., Laughlin, P., & Barchiesi, A. (1985). Nursing home care as an alternative to psychiatric hospitalization. *Archives of General Psychiatry, 42,* 544-551.

Linney, J. A. (1982). Alternative facilities for youth in trouble: Descriptive analysis of a strategically selected sample. In J. Handler & J. Zatz (Eds.), *Neither angels nor thieves: Studies in the deinstitutionalization of status offenders* (pp. 127-175). Washington, DC: National Academy Press.

Lyman, K. A. (1990). Staff stress and treatment of clients in Alzheimer's care: A comparison of medical and non-medical day care programs. *Journal of Aging Studies, 4,* 61-79.

Maloney, N., & Bowman, R. (1982). *Riverview Hospital Social Learning Program: Description and evaluation* (Project Report). Port Coquitlam, Vancouver, British Columbia: Riverview Hospital, Department of Psychology.

Manning, N. (1989). *The therapeutic community movement: Charisma and routinisation.* London: Routledge.

McCarthy, J., & Nelson, G. (1991). An evaluation of supportive housing for current and former psychiatric patients. *Hospital and Community Psychiatry, 42,* 1254-1256.

Moos, R. H. (1981). Environmental choice and control in community care settings for older people. *Journal of Applied Social Psychology, 11,* 23-43.

Moos, R. H. (1988a). Assessing the program environment: Implications for program evaluation and design. In K. J. Conrad & C. Roberts-Gray (Eds.), *New directions for program evaluation: Evaluating program environments* (Vol. 40, pp. 7-23). San Francisco: Jossey-Bass.

Moos, R. H. (1988b). *Community-Oriented Programs Environment Scale manual* (2nd ed.). Palo Alto, CA: Consulting Psychologists Press.

Moos, R. H. (1989). *Ward Atmosphere Scale manual* (2nd ed.). Palo Alto, CA: Consulting Psychologists Press.

Moos, R. H. (1994). *The Social Climate Scales: A user's guide* (2nd ed.). Palo Alto, CA: Consulting Psychologists Press.

Moos, R. H., David, T. G., Lemke, S., & Postle, E. (1984). Coping with an intra-institutional relocation: Changes in resident and staff behavior patterns. *The Gerontologist, 24,* 495-502.

Moos, R. H., & Lemke, S. (1980). Assessing the physical and architectural features of sheltered care settings. *Journal of Gerontology, 35,* 571-583.

Moos, R. H., & Lemke, S. (1983). Assessing and improving social-ecological settings. In E. Seidman (Ed.), *Handbook of social intervention* (pp. 143-162). Beverly Hills, CA: Sage.

Moos, R. H., & Lemke, S. (1984). Supportive residential settings for older people. In I. Altman, M. P. Lawton, & J. F. Wohlwill (Eds.), *Elderly people and the environment* (pp. 159-190). New York: Plenum.

Moos, R. H., & Lemke, S. (1985). Specialized living environments for older people. In J. E. Birren & K. W. Schaie (Eds.), *Handbook of the psychology of aging* (2nd ed., pp. 864-889). New York: Van Nostrand Reinhold.

Moos, R. H., & Lemke, S. (1992a). *Multiphasic Environmental Assessment Procedure: A user's guide.* Palo Alto, CA: Center for Health Care Evaluation, Department of Veterans Affairs and Stanford University Medical Centers.

Moos, R. H., & Lemke, S. (1992b). *Physical and Architectural Features Checklist manual.* Palo Alto, CA: Center for Health Care Evaluation, Department of Veterans Affairs and Stanford University Medical Centers.

Moos, R. H., & Lemke, S. (1992c). *Policy and Program Information Form manual.* Palo Alto, CA: Center for Health Care Evaluation, Department of Veterans Affairs and Stanford University Medical Centers.

Moos, R. H., & Lemke, S. (1992d). *Rating Scale manual.* Palo Alto, CA: Center for Health Care Evaluation, Department of Veterans Affairs and Stanford University Medical Centers.

Moos, R. H., & Lemke, S. (1992e). *Resident and Staff Information Form manual.* Palo Alto, CA: Center for Health Care Evaluation, Department of Veterans Affairs and Stanford University Medical Centers.

Moos, R. H., & Lemke, S. (1992f). *Sheltered Care Environment Scale manual.* Palo Alto, CA: Center for Health Care Evaluation, Department of Veterans Affairs and Stanford University Medical Centers.

Moos, R. H., & Lemke, S. (1994). *Group residences for older adults: Physical features, policies, and social climate.* New York: Oxford University Press.

Moos, R. H., Lemke, S., & Clayton, J. (1983). Comprehensive assessment of residential programs: A means of facilitating evaluation and change. *Interdisciplinary Topics in Gerontology, 17,* 69-83.

Moos, R. H., Lemke, S., & David, T. G. (1987). Priorities for design and management in residential settings for the elderly. In V. Regnier & J. Pynoos (Eds.), *Housing the aged: Design directives and policy considerations* (pp. 179-205). New York: Elsevier.

Mowbray, C. T., Greenfield, A., & Freddolino, P. P. (1992). An analysis of treatment services provided in group homes for adults labeled mentally ill. *Journal of Nervous and Mental Disease, 180,* 551-559.

Mulvey, E. P., Linney, J. A., & Rosenberg, M. S. (1987). Organizational control and treatment program design as dimensions of institutionalization in settings for juvenile offenders. *American Journal of Community Psychology, 15,* 321-335.

Nelson, G., & Earls, M. (1986). An action-oriented assessment of the housing and social support needs of long-term psychiatric clients. *Canadian Journal of Community Mental Health, 5,* 19-30

Netten, A. (1991-1992). A positive experience? Assessing the effect of the social environment on demented elderly residents of local authority homes. *Social Work and Social Sciences Review, 3,* 46-62.

Netten, A. (1992). *A positive environment? Physical and social influences on people with senile dementia in residential care.* Brookfield, VT: Ashgate.

Oberle, K., Wry, J., & Paul, P. (1988). *The relationship between environment, anxiety and post-operative recovery.* Alberta, Canada: University of Alberta Hospitals, Department of Nursing.

Orchowsky, S. J. (1982). Person-environment interaction in nursing homes for the elderly (Doctoral dissertation, Virginia Commonwealth University, Charlottesville, 1982). *Dissertation Abstracts International, 43,* 1240B.

Perkins, R. E., King, S. A., & Hollyman, J. A. (1989). Resettlement of old long-stay psychiatric patients: The use of the private sector. *British Journal of Psychiatry, 155,* 233-238.

Peters, H. J. M., & Boerma, L. H. (1982). *Onderzoek naar het leefklimaat in verpleeghuizen: Samenvatting van een vooronderzoek.* Nijmegen, The Netherlands: Netherlands Institute for Gerontology, Vakgroep Sociale Geneeskunde.

Peters, H. J. M., & Boerma, L. H. (1983). Leefklimaat in verpleeghuizen: Resultaat van een vooronderzoek. *Nederlands Tijdschrift Voor Sociale Gezondheidszorg, 61,* 278-279.

Phillips, C. J., & Henderson, A. S. (1991). The prevalence of depression among Australian nursing home residents: Results using draft ICD-10 and DSM-III-R criteria. *Psychological Medicine, 21,* 739-748.

Philp, I., Mutch, W. J., Devaney, J., & Ogston, S. (1989). Can quality of life of old people in institutional care be measured? *Journal of Clinical and Experimental Gerontology, 11,* 11-19.

Porter, R., & Watson, P. (1985). Environment: The healing difference. *Nursing Management, 16,* 19-24.

Ramian, K. (1987). The resident oriented nursing home: A new dimension in the nursing home debate: Emphasis on living rather than nursing. *Danish Medical Bulletin* (Special Suppl. Ser. No. 5), 89-93.

Rovins, G. (1990). Exploring the environmental effectiveness of normalization principles for older persons with developmental disabilities. *Adult Residential Care Journal, 4,* 37-49.

Sewell, F., & Lethaby, A. (1990). *Auckland homes for the elderly: Environmental quality and programmes.* Auckland, New Zealand: University of Auckland, Department of Community Health.

Sewell, F., & Marquis, C. (1989). *Quality and diversity of aged care institutions: A survey of Auckland hospitals.* Auckland, New Zealand: Department of Community Health, University of Auckland.

Shadish, W. R., Orwin, R. G., Silver, B. G., & Bootzin, R. R. (1985). The subjective well-being of mental patients in nursing homes. *Evaluation and Program Planning, 8,* 239-250.

Smith, G. C., & Whitbourne, S. K. (1990). Validity of the Sheltered Care Environment Scale. *Psychology and Aging, 5,* 228-235.

Smothers, B. (1987). The relationships among patient functional behaviors, patient characteristics, staff practices, and social climate in a psychiatric hospital (Doctoral dissertation, University of Maryland, College Park, 1986). *Dissertation Abstracts International, 48,* 1930B.

Spinner, B. J. H. (1986). Nursing home staff training in a modified aging microcosm module: Social climate and attitude change as perceived by residents and staff (Doctoral dissertation, University of Mississippi, 1985). *Dissertation Abstracts International, 46,* 3830A.

Stein, S., Linn, M. W., & Stein, E. M. (1987). Patients and staff assess social climate of different quality nursing homes. *Comprehensive Gerontology, 1,* 41-46.

Stevens, G., & Featherman, D. L. (1981). A revised socioeconomic index of occupational status. *Social Science Research, 10,* 364-395.

Svensson, T. (1984). *Aging and environment: Institutional aspects* (Linkoping Studies in Education, Vol. 21). Linkoping, Sweden: Linkoping University.

Thomas, T. (1989). *Admission into homes for the aged: A study in stress and coping.* Melbourne, Australia: Royal Melbourne Institute of Technology, Department of Social Science.

Thompson, B., & Swisher, M. (1983). An assessment, using the Multiphasic Environmental Assessment Procedure (MEAP), of a rural life-care residential center for the elderly. *Journal of Housing for the Elderly, 1,* 41-56.

Timko, C. (1995). Policies and services in residential substance abuse programs: Comparisons with psychiatric programs. *Journal of Substance Abuse, 7,* 43-59.

Timko, C. (1996). Physical characteristics of residential psychiatric programs: Organizational determinants and patient outcomes. *American Journal of Community Psychology, 24,* 173-192.

Timko, C., & Moos, R. H. (1989). Choice, control, and adaptation among elderly residents of sheltered care settings. *Journal of Applied Social Psychology, 19,* 636-655.

Timko, C., & Moos, R. H. (1990). Determinants of interpersonal support and self-direction in group residential facilities. *Journal of Gerontology: Social Sciences, 45,* S184-S192.

Timko, C., & Moos, R. H. (1991a). Assessing the quality of residential programs: Methods and applications. *Adult Residential Care Journal, 5,* 113-129.

Timko, C., & Moos, R. H. (1991b). A typology of social climates in group residential facilities for older people. *Journal of Gerontology: Social Sciences, 46,* S160-S169.

Timko, C., Nguyen, A. Q., Williford, W. O., & Moos, R. H. (1993). Quality of care and outcomes of chronic mentally ill patients in hospitals and nursing homes. *Hospital and Community Psychiatry, 44,* 241-246.

van Weert, N., & Beuken, N. (1987). *Leefklimaat in verpleeghuizen en verzorgingstehuizen.* Nijmegen, The Netherlands: Instituut voor Toegepaste Sociale Wetenschappen.

Wadsworth, J. S., & Harper, D. C. (1988). Residential assessment of adults with moderate mental retardation. *Perceptual and Motor Skills, 66,* 922.

Wadsworth, J. S., & Harper, D. C. (1989). *Enhancing self-report assessment of adults with moderate retardation.* Iowa City: University of Iowa, College of Medicine, Division of Developmental Disabilities.

Wandersman, A., & Moos, R. H. (1981a). Assessing and evaluating residential environments: A sheltered living environments example. *Environment and Behavior, 13,* 481-508.

Wandersman, A., & Moos, R. H. (1981b). Evaluating sheltered living environments for mentally retarded people. In M. C. Haywood & J. R. Newbrough (Eds.), *Living environments for developmentally retarded persons* (pp. 251-273). Baltimore, MD: University Park Press.

Waters, J. E. (1980a). The social ecology of long-term care facilities for the aged: A case example. *Journal of Gerontological Nursing, 6,* 155-160.

Waters, J. E. (1980b). Systematic measures of ideal nursing homes: Planning and research prospects. *Aging and Leisure Living, 3,* 14-16.

Waters, J. E. (1981). Enriching the teaching of social gerontology through use of a social climate scale. *Gerontology and Geriatrics Education, 2,* 65-68.

Weissert, W. G., Elston, J. M., Bolda, E. J., Cready, C. M., Zelman, W. N., Sloane, P. D., Kalsbeek, W. D., Mutran, E., Rice, T. H., & Koch, G. G. (1989). Models of adult day care: Findings from a national survey. *The Gerontologist, 29,* 640-649.

Wells, L. M. (1990). Responsiveness and accountability in long-term care: Strategies for policy development and empowerment. *Canadian Journal of Public Health, 81,* 382-385.

Wells, L. M., & Singer, C. (1988). Quality of life in institutions for the elderly: Maximizing well-being. *The Gerontologist, 28,* 266-269.

Wells, L. M., Singer, C., & Polgar, A. T. (1986). *To enhance quality of life in institutions: An empowerment model in long-term care: A partnership of residents, staff and families.* Toronto, Ontario, Canada: University of Toronto Press.

Willcocks, D., Peace, S., & Kellaher, L. (1987). *Private lives in public places: A research-based critique of residential life in local authority old people's homes.* London: Tavistock.

Wilson, J., & Kouzi, A. (1990). Quality of the residential environment in board-and-care homes for mentally and developmentally disabled persons. *Hospital and Community Psychiatry, 41,* 314-318.

Index

335

ABOUT THE AUTHORS

Rudolf H. Moos is Research Career Scientist and Director of the Center for Health Care Evaluation at the Veterans Affairs Palo Alto Heath Care System. He is also Professor of Psychiatry and Behavioral Sciences at the Stanford University School of Medicine. He received his training in clinical psychology from the Department of Psychology at the University of California, Berkeley and has conducted a program of research on residential and treatment environments and their impacts. He is the recipient of a number of honors including the Lazarsfeld Award of Evaluation Theory (1992) from the American Evaluation Association and the Distinguished Contribution Award from the Division of Community Psychology of the American Psychological Association.

Sonne Lemke is a Research Psychologist at the Center for Health Care Evaluation at the Veterans Affairs Palo Alto Health Care System. She received her training in developmental psychology from the Department of Psychology at the University of California, Berkeley, and in clinical psychology from the California School of Professional Psychology in Berkeley. She has overseen a long-term project to evaluate residential facilities for older people and coauthored a series of articles and a monograph on the characteristics of residential facilities and their impacts on older adults.